more peas please

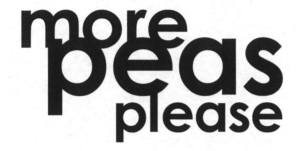

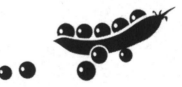

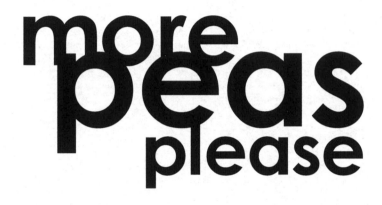

more peas please

SOLUTIONS FOR FEEDING FUSSY EATERS

KATE DI PRIMA & DR JULIE CICHERO

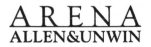

ARENA
ALLEN&UNWIN

First published in 2009

Arena Books, an imprint of
Allen & Unwin
83 Alexander Street
Crows Nest NSW 2065
Australia
Phone: (61 2) 8425 0100
Fax: (61 2) 9906 2218
Email: info@allenandunwin.com
Web: www.allenandunwin.com

Cataloguing-in-Publication details are available
from the National Library of Australia
www.librariesaustralia.nla.gov.au

ISBN 978 1 74175 715 6

Internal design by Emily O'Neill
Set in 12/16 pt Bembo by Midland Typesetters, Australia

FSC

Mixed Sources
Product group from well-managed
forests and other controlled sources

Cert no. SGS-COC-3047
www.fsc.org
© 1996 Forest Stewardship Council

The paper this book is printed on is certified by the © 1996 Forest
Stewardship Council A.C. (FSC). SOS holds FSC chain of custody
SGS-COC-3047. The FSC promotes environmentally responsible,
socially beneficial and economically viable management of the
world's forests.

Printed and bound in Australia by The SOS Print + Media Group.

10 9 8 7 6 5 4 3 2

Contents

List of tables

List of recipes

Acknowledgements

I would like to thank the following people without whom this book would not have been possible.

To my family: Jack and Rosie, you have been my inspiration and taught me that motherhood is the ultimate reward, thank you for all the challenges but—most of all—all the cuddles; my husband, Paul, who supported the many hours of writing and whipped up beautiful meals when the cupboard was bare.

To the patients and families who I have encountered through my practices and who have enriched my paediatric work.

To my wonderful colleague and inspirational writing buddy, Julie. Thank you for the journey and helping me to piece the fussy-eating puzzle together.

To Jo Paul, who went out on a limb for us.

Kate di Prima

This book is a culmination of many experiences, chance conversations and opportunities. I am grateful to my generous colleagues and researchers for sharing their wisdom, and to patients and their families who have taught me so much. Thank you to friends and family who shared their support, dinnertime triumphs and horror stories. Kate, thank you for the sore cheeks from laughter and the best fun I have ever had writing and learning about food! Most especially I wish to thank my family: to my husband, Jonathan, for his never-ending love and riotous good humour and to our children, Elliot, Phoebe and Xavier for your love, great company, cuddles at 5 a.m. at the computer and living the food adventure with me. Finally a huge thank you to all the fabulous folk at Allen & Unwin—you are wonderful people to work with!

Dr Julie Cichero

Introduction

To make a 'fuss' (noun): an agitated protest

'Fussy' (adjective): whining and fretting; hard to please; worrying about details

'Fussy eaters' are often described as children who refuse to try a new food at least half the time. Some parents would volunteer to swim shark-infested waters before subjecting themselves to yet another night of arguments about what their children will or won't eat. Chat to parents at a barbecue, family lunch, school pick-up zone or swimming carnival and you will hear someone talk about the fussy eater in their family. 'They'll eat fruit, but what do you do about the vegetables? Is it okay not to have the vegetables?', 'Mealtimes at our house are a cross between the noise on the floor of the stock exchange and someone leaving the 4-year-old in charge of traffic control at a busy intersection', 'I am so exhausted by the time I get home from work, I don't feel like fighting with the kids about dinner!'. Does any of this sound familiar? If it does, you are not alone. The overwhelming majority of parents are stressed about their children's eating habits, and about one-third of parents are concerned that their children are not eating enough. As parents of school-aged children ourselves, trust us when we say we hear you; we know what you're going through!

One of the first words we hear our children utter (after 'mum', 'dad' and 'ta') is 'no', coupled with a vigorous side-to-side shaking of the head. Most parents report that at six months of age their children slept well, played happily and ate anything that was put in front of them. Some time after that, and it does vary from child to child, they clamped their lips shut when offered their favourite foods or, worse, hurled the bowl off the highchair. The age of food fussiness has arrived. For parents, the two most difficult phases in a child's life to deal with are sleep issues and fussy eating practices—the latter lasting up to a number of years.

Somewhere between 18 months and two years of age your child enters a time of confidence, exploration and assertiveness. Many parents also deal with defiance, stubbornness and yes . . . fussiness! The word 'no' becomes the flavour of the month. It is used regularly to try to communicate with you, especially when it comes to the food that they want.

> 'No' means 'I don't want *that*'
> 'No' means 'I want the other one but I don't know what it is called'
> 'No' means 'I don't like that, although I did yesterday'
> 'No' means 'I don't know what that is'
> 'No' means 'I just don't know what I want'
> And 'No' means 'Just because!'

Communication between the two of you can become a complex game of charades. When you finally discover what it is they want, the treasured food becomes one of the few staples or 'favourites' that you continuously offer. Children then have an irritating habit of suddenly changing their mind at the most inconvenient time. Although they've been happy to eat porridge for the past three months, today and henceforth, porridge is now a banned substance. You are left to begin a frantic search, to again replace the once favourite food. You wake up one day to find that your little one has, slowly and stealthily over time, whittled their diet down to a grand total of five or so foods. Now there is no guarantee that these same foods will also satisfy their dietary requirements. So begins the daily struggle, first with your child and then with your conscience about the foods that are eaten in your house.

Parents want what is best for their child. They worry about whether their children are getting enough nutrition for growth and brain development, or getting enough iron and calcium for their immune system and bone development. Often parents know what it is they should be feeding their children. But there is this gaping chasm between knowing what children should eat, and actually getting them to eat healthy foods. Most parents aim to cross the chasm, however, without a safety net and with only a rickety bridge of knowledge, many turn back, dejected and disenchanted. Many parents see their child's eating inventory as a reflection of their parenting skills—the 'parent report-card', so to speak. Parents can skulk under the radar for years and to the outside world everything looks fine. Problems usually become 'urgent' once children start school, and the thought of lunchboxes, sleep-overs and school camps looms.

Parents and caregivers have told us that they are exhausted by the untouched lunchbox, or dread the nightly dinner ritual of arguments, tears and wasted food. For many it is easier to just give in, and serve up the same 'liked foods' everyday and hope their children grow out of it. Research shows us that many of our eating habits are well-ingrained by four years of age. It is only on entering early adulthood that most people become more adventurous about food. So the fact is, about 80 per cent of adults do *eventually* grow out of very fussy food tendencies. Just look around your office or social group. There aren't many adults still on plain white pasta and cheese, or Vegemite sandwiches with the crusts cut off. So somewhere between 12 months and 30 years of age, people become more inquisitive and open to trying things. Thankfully, you don't have to wait till your children are 30! *Anyone* can learn to try and enjoy new foods when given the right information and a set of realistic expectations.

In times gone by grandparents and neighbours would have helped parents to navigate their way through the maze of helping children to eat well. Times have changed. Many families now have two working parents, and grandparents who live close by are a scarce commodity. Mothers' groups and playgroups have been lifesaving for many new mums and dads who feel encouraged that other parents are dealing with similar issues to themselves. However, it can also be very stressful if children around the same age are achieving certain milestones before your little one. It is important to remember that children develop at a rate that is 'just right' for them. Take learning to walk, for example. Some little ones are up on their pins at ten months, whilst others are quite happy to sit tight until well over a year; however, they all walk by the time they are at school. There is a similar process to experimenting with foods.

Some toddlers are great eaters, consuming everything and anything that is given to them, whereas others would survive on mashed banana and yoghurt until they leave home. Some fussy eaters avoid whole groups of food. Others won't move from blended food without gagging on lumps, and then you have little ones who won't eat anything if it is covered in sauce. Believe it or not, there really is a phase of 'typical food fussiness'. How we, as parents, manage this phase has a huge impact on how children emerge on the other side. Overlapping with the terrible twos, this age is particularly tricky as children are also just learning language. Some frustrations are borne simply from communication breakdowns. Some children have had limited exposure to new foods; you need to try a new food 10–15 times before the brain stops labelling it as 'new'! Many times it is not the taste of the food but the texture of food that puts children off. For some children the timing of meals is off and their hunger cycles are running out of sync with the grown-ups in the family. Some children have not yet developed their chewing skills. Provide a child who has limited chewing skills with a piece of meat, and you can be sure that it will be spat out again. This is a safety mechanism designed so that children do not choke on food that has been inadequately masticated. There are medically related issues that affect children's desire to eat, such as constipation, reflux, or enormous tonsils and adenoids. The body is cleverly designed and sometimes there are sound reasons for food refusal. While there may be many reasons why your child is 'fussy', you can feel like you are constantly hitting your head against a brick wall whilst you battle on trying to change your child's eating habits.

Without realising it, *we*, as parents, can also make a fuss about food. We break out the party streamers when children eat vegetables, and paint our faces and declare war when food is left on the dinner plate. Learning to try new foods is a process, much like going from rolling to crawling, to walking and running. Sometimes we forget that we are 'experts' at eating. We are used to seeing different foods because we've been exposed to them for years and years. Take your child to the zoo and watch their wonder and amazement at the different animals. For parents, an elephant is an elephant is an elephant. For your child, it is an incredible being with a strange-looking nose, wiry hair and lots of wrinkles. Follow the analogy and for a grown-up, a grape is a grape is a grape. For your child, it is smooth and dry on the outside and wet and squishy on the inside—talk about a mind-trip!

We believe that one of the keys to making sure your child's diet is balanced is to encourage them to consume a wide variety of foods and textures. This is exactly what we have been doing for the past ten years when helping parents and carers with their fussy eaters. In order to feel confident about your food choices and your household rules, we believe that you need some important information. It is essential that you know:

- what it is that constitutes a good diet
- how to help children develop good chewing skills so that they are not stuck with a lifetime of soft foods
- when to stop making separate 'kids' meals' and 'adult meals'
- what quantities children eat and how these portion sizes are different to what adults eat
- how to help children develop skills for trying new foods
- the time and patience it takes to develop new eating habits
- some basics about how the body works and grows and that these factors definitely affect your child's appetite and eating patterns
- that children are growing and hence are changing, whereas we have stopped growing, so our food experiences are different to theirs
- what motivates children to eat food and which tactics backfire and turn them off
- how to react when foods are rejected
- how to pack a mean lunchbox
- how to take the fuss out of the dinnertime fiasco, from children in highchairs to teenagers.

In short, we'd like you to know how to welcome our little foreigners and induct them into our tribal eating customs. As parents we feel the weight of that enormous responsibility. Our reactions to how and what our children eat are critical.

HOW WILL THIS BOOK HELP YOU?

This book is as relevant to new parents who are just embarking on the world of solids, as it is to parents of teenagers. In fact, many families have children at different ages and stages. The key is knowing how to improve their diet and gaining the knowledge and skills to do so. *More Peas Please* is an easy-to-follow guide to help you understand why children are fussy and help you with strategies to improve your child's eating habits. You will find that some of the chapters are specific to children at particular ages or stages in life. From how to prevent fussy eating from taking up residence in your house, to dealing with its aftermath, there are chapters to address all of the common issues. You will also find most chapters have universal relevance, such as 'What is a good diet?', 'Hiding vegetables in cakes. Is it worth it?', 'The "rules of engagement": Rules at mealtimes' and 'Tips for shopping, cooking, lunchboxes and others'.

The step-by-step chapters will show you how to get children to try something new and will also show you what foods and meals to use when whole food groups are being avoided. Chapters covered include: developmental stages and what children should be eating at certain ages; surviving the age of fussy eating; and medical reasons for food refusal. There are valuable sections on defiance and causes of fussiness to help you understand how to tackle food avoidance. There are sections on novel ways of explaining the value of different foods in terms that children can relate to, and useful tips for developing new habits. There are also some foolproof recipes to ensure that you are maximising your child's nutrition. In short, it is like having a dietitian and a feeding and swallowing specialist at your fingertips!

IT'S TIME TO STOP THE FUSS

True to the importance of food in our everyday life, this book was shaped and moulded through many discussions in a coffee shop. Staff often asked when the next meeting was and we fondly looked forward to our 'next instalment'. Close your eyes and you can smell the aroma of coffee and hear the sounds of laughter as we discussed our own dinnertime anecdotes and stories. On a serious note, though, this book is very important. The single greatest gift that we can give to our children is for them to live longer than ourselves. Certainly we don't want their life expectancy to shrink. We have a window of opportunity to help children develop the habits that they will need for a lifetime. Children's physical and cognitive growth depends on what they eat. At no other time in their life is it so urgent that we get it right. Thankfully, it is never too late to start developing new habits. Even fussy adults can learn to eat new foods using the advice contained within these pages. We hope that a book like *More Peas Please* will be your 'food bible', to have on hand for children of any age. It will help you fill in the missing foods, trudge your way through the difficult times of the 'age of fussiness', but most importantly give you the confidence that you are giving your child the best start in life. Enjoy, and for goodness sake . . . stop the fuss!

Developmental stages of eating

Many books provide information on the first few spoonfuls of solids on days one to three and then leave parents to wander the wilderness of transitioning from exclusive milk feeds to milk feeds plus solids on their own. Just like breastfeeding, many people assume that introducing solids is a simple and straightforward affair. As parents ourselves we know that no two children are the same. However, there are some foundation guidelines that certainly help. Over the next few sections we will show you how to introduce solids, how to move on to lumpy textures, soft foods, finger foods and 'grown-up people' foods. We will provide you with information on why it is important to introduce solids at around six months of age and why children gag.

This chapter is the mechanical guide to feeding. It will help you to understand the way a child learns to eat. Yes—*learns* to eat! We are all aware of how a child learns to walk. Children start by having the strength and balance to sit. They progress to movement via crawling. They learn to balance and stand. Then there's furniture cruising and finally walking! There are also steps to learning to eat. And much like learning to walk, they need time and practice. This chapter will also provide you with useful cues on reading your child's developmental feeding age rather than their chronological age and choosing foods of the right food texture for their skill level.

SIX MONTHS—INTRODUCING FIRST SOLIDS

The World Health Organization recommends that solids are introduced from six months of age.[1] In days gone by, first solids were introduced at four months and you may still come across some paediatricians who have specific reasons for recommending this slightly earlier introduction (see also Chapter 5, 'Medical reasons for food refusal'). Until the age of six months children are completely reliant on breast milk or formula. At six months of age children's bodies and muscles have grown and developed sufficiently to begin to try the tricky process of eating. Why tricky? Because we use 26 different muscles to eat and swallow. We also have to coordinate our eating and breathing. We all hold our breath for a moment while we swallow so that food and liquid goes down 'the right way'. Prior to about six months of age children just do not have the strength and control to manage solids. They need to have sufficient body strength to keep their head and body stable. They also need good strength and control of their mouth muscles to safely manage solids.

Many parents quietly mark off the calendar for the day when their child turns six months with the expectation that any sleep, or irritability issues, will be solved by this magic introduction of solid food. Time to 'burst the bubble'. First solids are for practice. Until this point in time, 'food' has been delivered to the very back of the baby's mouth, making it easy for receptors there to trigger a swallow. These 'solids' are in fact a thickish liquid and are placed onto the middle of the tongue. Your baby now has to learn to move it to the back of the mouth; to the right spot for it to be swallowed. So, first solids provide them with practice at *manipulating* food and *moving* it to the right spot. If on day one you get a quarter of a teaspoon in over three attempts, you've done well. Realistic expectations are important. Your baby is not going to eat even half a cup of puree on day one or anytime soon thereafter. Initially, your baby may not even realise what you are trying to do with the spoon!

First solids are also introduced at six months to reduce the risk of food allergies and intolerances. Research studies have shown that children who are introduced to solids earlier than four to six months have a higher risk of developing food allergies or intolerances.[2] The baby's digestive system is also too immature to cope with food other than breast milk or formula.

Setting the stage

The grand day arrives and you are ready to start introducing your little one to solids. Until this point in time your baby has learned that feeling hungry equals sucking. You are now going to teach them that hunger can also be appeased by a different means. Unfortunately, a baby who is hungry for their breastfeed or bottle-feed is unlikely to be interested in a spoon. Mid-morning seems to be a good time of day to start solids. Early in the morning and after a good four or more hours sleep, nothing is going to come between your baby and their milk! Solids at the end of the day when baby is tired are also less likely to be successful.

Use a small flat spoon, something even smaller than a teaspoon if possible. The spoon is like a miniature bowl. A bowl that is flat will hold a small amount and slide off fairly easily. A deep bowl means that you have to use your top lip to pull the material out of the bowl. Help baby with this new experience by using a small spoon with a flat bowl. As they become more experienced with taking food from a spoon, you can move on to different types of spoons. As they grow and their oral cavity becomes larger, they will be able to manage the amount that a child-size or adult-size spoon provides them. Look at the size of your child's mouth and the size of the spoon and ensure that they are an appropriate match. Many preschoolers are still 'growing into' adult-size breakfast spoons.

Seating and starting

Ensure your baby is sitting up and well-supported. Investment in a good highchair will stand you in good stead. Ensure your baby feels safe and secure. A child who feels unstable and about to fall over will not be interested in eating. Feeding your baby so that they can see your face is really important. They can see you open your mouth as you bring the spoon to their lips and see you smile as they take their first taste. It is normal for babies to pull faces. For the entirety of their life they have been having breast milk or formula and here you are giving them something quite different in taste and texture to this. They may be surprised! It may take as many as ten to 15 little tastes for them to get used to new flavours and textures. On day one you might get just three little tastes in. Step it up by about a teaspoon each day so that by about day eight your child will be having two tablespoons of solids. Whilst this might not sound like much to us, remember that they have little tummies. For each new taste, allow about three days to see how they take to it and whether they have any reactions.

What do first solids look like?

First solids have the thickness or consistency of smooth runny custard. Up until now your baby has been having breast milk or formula that is more of a liquid consistency. With the extra manipulation required to move the food to the back of the mouth, it is important that the food does not move too quickly and accidentally 'go down the wrong way'. Foods or drinks that 'go down the wrong way' are actually going into the airway. Most of us cough when this happens to remove these substances. Now, there is a fine line between runny, thick and sticky. It is important that this new substance is *not* sticky, like mashed potato, for example. Sticky foods need tongue strength to release the sticky substance from the tongue surface and push it towards the back of the mouth. Runny purees are thicker than normal liquids, but are slippery, making it easier to move them to the back of the mouth. They are smooth and don't hold their shape on a spoon. Placed on a plate, spoonfuls will bleed into each other rather than hold their own shape. In short, they are great for practising the movement that is needed to move food from the front of the mouth to the back of the mouth for it to be swallowed.

Runny purees can be suckled from the spoon. Until now baby has been used to sucking to gain food. These first solids mark a transition from sucking to more controlled movement patterns necessary for the different textures of food they will meet as they get older. The bridge, though, is often a 'suckling' from the spoon, as we might do with a thick soup. It is recommended that first solids be served at body temperature, just the same as their milk. Once your little one is managing this runny texture, you can thicken it up to the consistency of a smooth yoghurt or thick custard. In the supermarkets this may be called 'Stage One or First Foods' (see also Table 4).

How do I go about introducing solids?

As mentioned above, for the first few weeks, first solids are for practice and learning. Your little one will gain very little nutritionally from these experiences. They remain reliant on breast milk or formula. In order to reduce the likelihood of an allergy or intolerance, first foods are generally introduced in the following order:

- iron fortified rice cereal
- pureed fruits or vegetables
- pureed protein foods (e.g. meat, chicken, fish).

Aim to stick with one food for about three days before introducing the next one. Baby cereals are a good constant because of their iron content. Iron from solids is essential from six months of age. You can provide your little one with variety in the different foods you offer. Avoid mixing foods together in the early days. This makes it easier to spot a reaction if one is going to occur. Now, this is where the explanation can cause confusion. Baby can have apple and pumpkin on the same day, just not mixed together if it is the first time they have had either the pumpkin or the apple. For a practical example, please see the table below for a guide to introducing solids.

Table 1: **Guide to introducing solids**

Day 1	Iron fortified cereal (mix 1 teaspoon with approx. 1 tablespoon of breast milk, formula or cooled boiled water)	Offer 1 teaspoon of mixture.
Days 2–3	Iron-fortified cereal (as above)	As above, increase to 2 teaspoons, as tolerated.
Day 4	Iron-fortified cereal (as above)	Increase to 3 teaspoons, as tolerated.
Days 5–10	Iron-fortified cereal (as above)	Increase amount by 1 teaspoon per day (max. of 2 tablespoon per day).
Day 11	Iron-fortified cereal plus fruit pureed until smooth and slippery	6–7 teaspoons of rice plus 1–2 teaspoons of fruit puree. Don't mix together.
Days 12–14	Iron-fortified cereal plus fruit puree	Increase to 3 teaspoons of fruit puree. Use same fruit puree for 3 days before progressing to new fruit/ vegetable. Once tolerated for 3 days, puree can be mixed in with cereal.

Day 15	Continue to introduce new purees (fruit, vegetable, protein)	Keep 'new' food separate for first few days each time. After this time 'new' foods can be mixed with foods already tried. Keep 'new' foods small in quantity to begin with (e.g. 1 tablespoon).

Julie distinctly remembers coming home one day to find her husband happily feeding their daughter Phoebe pureed pumpkin. She had tried this herself on a number of occasions with no success and yet here she was happily opening her mouth wide for more. Julie's husband's explanation? Phoebe preferred him feeding her! Fine by Julie! About half an hour later he admitted that he had added about a teaspoon of pineapple juice to the pumpkin. While pureed fruits had been happily consumed, some vegetables, such as the pumpkin, were proving difficult. With the happy cherub having previously eaten pineapple juice with rice cereal there were no concerns about adverse reactions. The odd mixture of pineapple juice and pureed pumpkin proved to be a surprisingly successful combination.

We have heard mums say that they tried to introduce solids and it 'didn't go well' so they left it a couple of weeks before trying again. Again it didn't go well, and so they held off for another week or two, and suddenly we were seeing a 12–14-month-old who was purely breastfed or formula-fed. These children are at risk for lacking essential nutrients that are imperative for development of their brain, skin, immune system, metabolism and essential systems.

In addition, periods of critical development for oral skills are also being missed. Imagine picking up your child each time they looked distressed or frustrated at learning to crawl or walk. It is certainly easier from their point of view to be carried rather than to crawl. You may even enjoy the special bond and their need for you. But unless the child is exposed to trying, they will not establish or improve their skills. If the first 'feeding experience' does not go well, try it again the next day. Try at a different time of day. Consistency is imperative. Most babies do not like having their pooey nappy changed, but this doesn't mean you let them dictate the rules; you are in charge.

Keep feeding sessions short. You will only need about five minutes. Remember to keep smiling, to open your mouth and show your baby what it is you want them to do. Remember to give plenty of smiles and cuddles after each feeding session. This feeding business should be a happy time. If after two weeks of *daily* practice you are still experiencing difficulties, seek help. Do not delay. It will not get better by itself; in fact, it will get harder.

So, to summarise, around six months of age your baby will be having rice cereal. By about seven months of age your little one could also be having pureed fruit and pureed vegetables. Soon after, pureed protein foods (meat, chicken and fish) should be introduced for the all-important iron that's so necessary to brain development.

How do I know when they've had enough?

Approximately the first four weeks of solids is spent in the learning phase. In the first two weeks you may have worked your way up to about 1 tablespoon of food at mid-morning sandwiched between milk feeds. By the end of the third week you may have tried giving some solids after their morning milk feed as well as mid-morning or lunch. And by the fourth week you might be giving your little one solids after the morning milk feed, at around lunchtime and again at afternoon tea time for a total of 2–3 tablespoons of solids each day.

There is a delicate dance that is being played out. In addition to gradually introducing different tastes and flavours and gradually building up quantity, parents are also trying to figure out what the capacity of their child's tank is. Once your child is happy to have food given to them from the spoon and is actively engaged in the process, take your cues from your child. Lots of smiles each time your baby takes some food into their mouth increases the chance of them doing it again. Any face-pulling on your part because you are giving them pureed pumpkin, which may make your skin crawl, will likely have them showing the same response back to you. You are communicating! When they clamp their mouth shut or turn their head away, it may be their way of telling you 'I've had enough'.

There are a few other factors that will dictate how much a child will eat at mealtimes. Babies have little tummies—their portion-size needs are smaller than we think. The Stage One jar foods hold about one-quarter of a cup of pureed food. They also claim to be a single serve. If a baby starts solids at six months of age, they are unlikely to be managing a quarter of a cup of food until they are maybe six-and-a-half to seven months of age, all things going well. Keep your expectations of what they will eat realistic and listen to their cues. A predominance of milk means less interest in solids. Our job is to gradually change the balance over.

A baby who is unsettled because they are teething or who has a head cold will be less interested in eating. Keep offering solids, but make allowances for illness. On the other hand a baby who is very active and learning to crawl or who is stimulated by outings or learning to swim may, at times, have a larger appetite. Appetite will vary with activity levels in the same way that ours does. Respond accordingly.

Late introduction to solids—Why can't we just keep breastfeeding?

Evidence shows the many benefits of breast milk for infants. However, we have noticed a trend towards late introduction to solids. Some parents are delaying this introduction until ten months and beyond. While breast milk or formula remains the single most important element in a baby's diet to 12 months of age, there are important reasons for introducing solids at six months. As noted above, these first forays into solids are for tastes and practice. Children cannot progress to lumpy textures, finger foods and big-people foods without first having learned to deal with 'first solids'. They will only move through the progression of food textures if they have been given the opportunity to practise each step along the way. This early feeding practice exercises and shows the full skill of the tongue. This is an important early 'workout' for the tongue which has such a large role in learning to talk too.

Children will not suddenly refuse the breast because they are starting solids. The quantities that they start with are too small to have a large effect on milk consumption. The idea is to gradually shift the balance, so that by 12 months of age your little one will be having regular food and also still enjoy breastfeeding or drinking milk from a cup or bottle. So, when introduced with a good measure of commonsense, starting solids allows this gradual change in balance towards food, just the way that nature intended. If, however, there are any concerns about the adequacy or quantity of breast milk, this should be addressed as a separate issue. Discussions with a lactation consultant or your GP are advised.

Apart from an important introduction to oral development, the introduction to solids allows infants to continue to receive sufficient iron stores which are vital to brain development. During the last trimester, iron stores are laid down. Iron stores are critical for brain development and also have a role in the hunger cycle. The baby uses these iron stores during their first 4–6 months of life. The body does not produce iron, so the only way to add to the iron stores is via iron-rich foods. This is why first cereals are iron-fortified.

Gagging and vomiting

Why do children gag? And, let's face it, sometimes it can be pretty spectacular! There are physiological and developmental reasons why babies gag on solids, including purees. Contrary to popular belief, it is not because they don't like your cooking. Babies are born with the gag reflex being triggered from anywhere beyond the front quarter of the tongue. It is a protective reflex. Babies do not have the skills to remove objects with their fingers. They do not have the oral manipulation skills to chew food till it is soft and small enough to be swallowed. Nature has stepped in by installing an 'eject' mechanism before anything gets to the point of no return at the back of the tongue, where reflexes ordinarily trigger a swallowing reflex. This is a natural response in babies to eject items (food/buttons/toys) that could block their airway. Gagging occurs in older children when the piece of food they are trying to swallow is too large, or if the texture, taste or smell is unfamiliar or unpleasant.

By necessity this gag reflex has to be dampened to allow food to be introduced. This dampening process begins around six months of age, and the stimulus area for triggering the gag reflex moves to the back half of the tongue. Babies assist the dampening of the gag reflex by sucking on their fist, pushing their fingers into their mouths and sucking, or mouthing teething toys. Infants who are not readily able to get their hands up to their mouths may have a persistent and 'trigger-happy' gag reflex. An overzealous gag reflex can quickly and easily trigger its companion vomiting reflex.

Choking occurs when the child cannot physically breathe. Children who are choking will not be able to cry, and will be distressed and frightened. It is imperative that the food is removed from the mouth or throat using first-aid procedures to ensure that the child can breathe again.

To avoid gagging, when starting with first solids, bring the spoon to the lips and just into the mouth. Pushing the spoon too far into the mouth may cause your child to gag or vomit. Technique is important. Gagging and vomiting is not pleasant and a child will avoid this experience and the eating that goes with it if it happens too often. As you move on to lumpy textures, pressure on the gum ridges triggers another useful reflex, the biting reflex; this is the rudimentary beginning of chewing and munching (see the following section 'Seven to nine months—Introducing lumpy solids'). In short, gagging can just be some impressive feedback that you have gone too far or presented the child with too great a challenge for their current skill level.

Some infants may vomit when they have had too much. They may be so wrapped up in the experience of eating that they ignore their body's message to stop. Some babies, on the other hand, are seasoned 'chuckers'. These little ones often have a diagnosis of reflux. For the most part, it is thought that the introduction to solids will reduce problems associated with feeding for reflux-prone babies. Parents of reflux bubs, who continue to vomit after their introduction to solids, may wish to consider further investigations. In a very small proportion of cases, some babies may vomit due to food intolerance or food allergy. Reflux, food intolerances and allergies are covered in detail in Chapter 5, 'Medical reasons for food refusal'.

Introducing cup-drinking

Cup-drinking can be introduced from six months of age. This is a great time to start the practice they need, so that by the time they really need those cup-drinking skills, they look like a professional. Start your introduction to cup-drinking by expecting there to be some mess, some coughing and looks of surprise. During breastfeeding or bottle-feeding, infants have learned to groove their tongue to accommodate the breast or bottle teat. This is good practice for the tongue muscles to learn to create a little cup. With breast feeding or bottle-feeding, liquid is delivered directly to the back of the baby's mouth. They do not have to catch and control the liquid and guide it to the right spot. During early cup-drinking attempts the liquid quickly reaches the back of the tongue and escapes over into the throat. The throat is also the entry to the airway so some liquid is likely to end up in the airway because this system has not been given enough time or the right signals to protect itself. This is where the coughing and surprised looks come in. Children however, learn very quickly. A little bit of coughing will not hurt them and will help to teach them by consequence what happens if they rush the liquid into their mouth. You need to remain calm and reassure them so that they do not become anxious or distressed. Note also, persistent, violent coughing should be investigated.

You can introduce a spout cup as a transition from the breast or bottle to the cup, or move straight to an open cup. Sports water bottles are not recommended for children who are just learning to manage liquids. Spout cups can be made from a soft rubber. This variety often has a cross cut in the top so that as the child sucks, the hole opens to allow the liquid to flow. Other spouts are made from hard plastic and have two or three holes in the top to allow unrestricted flow when the cup is tipped.

Valved spout cups have become very popular. The suction required to gain any liquid from these devices is extraordinary (try it for yourself!). This often results in children attempting to take sips from the valved cup but abandoning it because it is just too difficult. Valved cups were designed for the convenience of parents to minimise spills. They do not have any benefits for the child and, as noted before, can be detrimental in terms of teaching them to drink from a spout cup. You may choose to buy a valved spout cup for travel and when you are out and about, simply remove the valve when it is time for the child to drink and replace it when it's time to travel to minimise spills.

Little cups work best for little mouths. A little plastic medicine cup or a hard plastic shot glass is ideal. For open-cup drinking and spout-cup drinking, you are in charge of the liquid flow while your baby has their learner plates on. They have no concept of how fast liquid flows or what a good mouthful size is—this is the stuff of funny home videos. Hold the cup to their mouth and tip it up so that a very small amount initially goes onto their lips and into their mouth. It is okay if they clamp their jaws on the cup to help hold it steady. Stay calm and smile and provide encouragement. Close your lips in a slightly exaggerated way and pretend to swallow. You could expect: some liquid to dribble out of their mouth; for the first couple of mouthfuls to be swallowed and then the remainder forcefully spat back (to this a firm 'no' is required); coughing or looks of utter surprise. As with all things new, frequent opportunities to practise are important. But, sessions need to be really short so that children don't become fearful, frustrated or defiant. So try one or two sips, three or four times a day. Let your child take the lead and if they want more, provide more. When they want to stop, then finish up and provide lots of smiles and hugs so that they are more inclined to want to try it again next time. Always stop before the child becomes cranky. Before long they will be reaching for your cup as you drink! Water is the best liquid to put into either a spout cup or an open cup. For the breastfeed-a-holic bub, some expressed breast milk will work well initially too.

Lose the dummy, lose the bottle

The length of time a child spends with a bottle or dummy seems to have got longer over the past 20-odd years. Maybe the boom in sports bottles has somehow made the bottle seem normal. Babies' main source of nutrition comes from breast or bottle till

12 months of age. By this time babies should be taking solids and be adept at drinking from a spout cup and/or an open cup. Retaining a bottle delays this process. It also significantly increases the chances of dental problems. Bubs put to bed with a bottle in their mouth, or who wander around with a bottle hanging from their mouth, are bathing brand new baby teeth in liquid, which puts them at risk of cavities.

Babies who suck on a dummy have a major impediment for learning how to speak. Language delays can be common in children with long-term dummy use. If your little one needs a dummy to help them settle for sleep, then keep it just for this purpose. Avoid the temptation to use it as a plug for when they might be crying. Aim to start transitioning out the bottles and dummies when they are 12 months of age. Some will manage fine without a fight, whereas others will hang on for dear life. The aim is for them to be dummy- and bottle-free by their second birthday. The constant sucking pressure also affects the formation of bones inside their mouth and might cost you a small fortune in orthodontic bills to have it rectified. It is worth the time and effort now.

SEVEN TO NINE MONTHS—INTRODUCING LUMPY SOLIDS

By this stage you will have a little person who has had a good month or more of practice with runny and smooth purees. They understand what the spoon is about and are keen to try food. Now is the time to introduce very small soft lumps to their food to help them learn to chew. It is really important that they learn to do this at seven to nine months of age even though children will not get all of their chewing teeth (molars or back teeth) until they are 12–24 months old.

There are muscles in the cheeks (masseter muscles) and up near the temples (temporalis muscles) that are important for chewing. They get stronger over time and with repeated use. Let's think back to that 'learning to walk' model. With smooth purees your baby has learned to crawl, this next step is learning to stand up. A baby who is learning to stand up will only stand for short periods of time because they are getting their balance and their muscles are getting stronger each time they practise. The same is true for lumpy solids. In learning to chew, they first need to recognise that there is a lump there. Lumps need to go to the gum ridges. Once on the gum ridges, there are sensors that tell the gums to 'munch' in an up–down pattern. This is the earliest form of chewing. With nice soft lumps, baby gets practice at the right action and the muscles slowly get stronger, allowing them to move on to foods that require more chewing and manipulation.

To start with, your baby will probably try to swallow the lumpy food straight down as they have with the puree. To start with, this may cause gagging. As noted above, the back of the tongue has a lot of sensors to alert the brain to elements that can cause a choking risk. Once the baby learns to break down the soft lumps, this is enough for the tongue sensors to relax and allow the food to be swallowed without the gagging.

Lumps can be introduced in a variety of ways. Food can be finely mashed rather than pureed smooth. Alternatively, you can add grated cheese or fine breadcrumbs to smooth puree to provide a soft lumpy texture. Mashed pieces of tinned fruit or soft fresh fruit can be added to purees. It is important that the lumps are very small and very soft to start with. For the first five days you may wish to have two bowls handy: one with smooth puree and one with lumpy puree. Start with the smooth puree and offer a couple of spoonfuls, and then offer a spoonful of the lumpy puree. Each spoonful of lumpy puree should have only one or two soft lumps in it to start with. Gradually move to having one smooth spoonful then one lumpy, and finally change it over so that all lumpy solids are provided. Once these soft lumps are managed well, the number of lumps can be increased. After a period of managing soft lumpy puree, slightly harder lumps can be tried. Slightly harder lumps include cooked rice and risoni pasta. Even once your baby is taking lumpy purees, smooth purees often still remain in the diet, in the form of yoghurts or custards. In the supermarkets, lumpy purees are often referred to as 'Stage Two or Second Foods'.

EIGHT TO TEN MONTHS—INTRODUCING MASHED, CHOPPED, SOFT FOODS AND FINGER FOODS

Let's go back to our 'walking analogy'. Your little one is now very capable of managing smooth textures and lumpy-textured purees—the walking equivalent of crawling and standing. Now it is time to learn to walk. By about 8–10 months of age, your child is also keen to hold food and swipe at the spoon. You may already have half the cutlery drawer out so that you still have a spoon in your hand for feeding your increasingly independent child. Now that soft lumps are managed well, it is time to move towards fork-mashed foods, finely chopped foods and soft foods. Fork-mashed foods will provide more opportunities for chewing practice. The pieces will be slightly larger and you may need to put in a little less so that your child can move the pieces around for adequate chewing.

Now, here's the trick to introducing finely chopped foods and soft finger foods. Try one or two pieces of grated cheese. Take these small pieces on your finger and pop them into the left or right side or your child's mouth on the lower gum ridges. Your child's jaw will start to move up and down. Particularly if you are doing a chewing action with your own jaw, then smiling and cooing encouragement. Watch carefully. You should be able to see their tongue move across to the side where you put the food. This is another important step for learning to chew. The tongue's job is to collect lumps and transport them over to the gums (and eventually the teeth) to be broken down to a consistency that is safe to swallow. By breaking tiny pieces off (think the size of biscuit crumbs), you are helping your child to learn how to manage lumps that are not encased in a puree. Once your child learns to manage these tiny bits, you can start to make the pieces a little bit bigger. Use the size of your child's thumbnail as a guide. Now you are giving them their first lessons in what will be a good 'bite size'.

Julie recently watched a mum hand half a pikelet to her 10-month-old. His first response was to mash it in his fist. He was enjoying the texture. She was dismayed—'See, see! He won't eat it.' Julie salvaged a small piece and popped it in on his left side, smiled and then pretended to chew, and behold, he started to chew. A few chews later and he had swallowed it down and was looking for more. The mum repeated the process with success. Within five minutes he had eaten the entire piece of pikelet. No gagging, no food throwing. It was the most finger food he had ever eaten. It was also the first time he had been actively taught what to do with pieces that were just the right size for his little mouth.

Foods that will work well at the lumpy solids and soft finger foods stage are included in the following table.

Emerging independence—Self-feeding and safe food textures

Once your little one can safely manage soft foods in little pieces, you can provide them with small amounts on their tray for them to self-feed. You can also progress to soft finger foods. These are also included in Table 2. You will notice that toast, but not bread, has been included in the table. Even though we tend to think of bread as soft, it actually isn't. Think about it—you can't fork-mash bread. You need quite a bit of chewing power to break down bread. Many babies who are provided with bread will suck it and use their saliva to soften it until little pieces or chunks become detached. They certainly don't chew it! It is a good

Table 2: **Stage Two foods and finger foods**

Pasta (e.g. risoni)
Rice
Tinned fruit (peach, apricot)
Fresh fruit (banana, mango, rockmelon)
Steamed vegetables pieces
Omelette
Mashed boiled eggs
Porridge
Grated cheese
Finely chopped ham or chicken
Soft mince (e.g. spaghetti sauce)
Fish rissoles
Soft mince meatballs
Soft biscuits (Scotch Finger biscuits, Clix biscuits, rice biscuits)
Cruskits
Wafers
Warm toast

Note: Ensure initial Stage Two foods are presented in small pieces—the size of an adult's little fingernail.

food to help build up their jaw muscle strength, but only once they are about 12 months of age, unless you can see that their chewing skills are very well-developed. Crustless toast is a modified introduction to bread. The heating process and the addition of a condiment to the heated bread, allowing it to seep in, softens the toast. Cruskits provide a good sandwich substitute at this stage. Although hard, these crispbreads dissolve very quickly when water or saliva is added to them. This reduces the choking risk, provided that pieces are kept small and children are not allowed to overstuff their mouths. Avocado, Vegemite, cream cheese and hommus can all be spread onto a Cruskit to provide an introduction to flavours and keep the Cruskit interesting.

Keep an eye on the textures you are offering. Have something easy, something manageable and something a little more challenging. If you only include challenging foods, your child is likely to refuse them. Think back to the development of those chewing muscles. Remember what your jaw feels like when you are eating a really crusty bread roll. It aches! If you are working too hard, you tend to give up. In children we see this as taking a couple of chews and then spitting the food out. Sometimes parents interpret this as the child not liking the taste of the food. In fact, the child may be telling us that they don't yet have the muscle strength to manage the texture. It's a bit like expecting a child to be able to pick up a 2 kg weight because they have arms, and we lift weights with our arms. Unless you step up slowly from smaller weights, you do not have the strength to perform with heavier weights. The same is true for the jaw muscles and their ability to manage harder-textured foods.

It is important to try something challenging in small spurts, and often. If you only provide the easy foods, then that is all they will learn to manage. We have seen 3-year-olds with a diet of solely smooth purees, custards and yoghurts because it was 'what they would take'. These children had poor chewing skills, but once they had learned to chew were more accepting of different textures. In the supermarkets, mashed foods and soft foods with more uneven texture may be called 'Stage Three' foods.

Learning to 'take a bite'

Children have no internal representation of what 'taking a bite' is all about. We say it and magically expect them to know what we are talking about. We may show them, but because the food chunk disappears into our mouth, the child does not see how big or small that chunk is. As a rough guide, use either your child's thumbnail size or your little finger's nail size as an appropriate guide to the size of a 'bite'. Using finger foods this size can teach your child an appropriate size for their mouth over a couple of days. You can then ask them to 'take a bite' and they should be better able to determine whether the chunk they have taken is okay for them. Try this activity with a soft food (e.g. banana) or a dissolvable food (e.g. shortbread biscuit). Once you're confident they've got the idea, you can progress to different food textures.

TWELVE TO 24 MONTHS—INTRODUCING 'GROWN-UP' FOOD (WITH SOME EXCLUSIONS)

With your child having progressed through the stages outlined above, they will be developmentally ready to start more 'grown-up' textured foods. By about 12 months of age, the average adult dinner can be served with minor modifications. In all cases, pieces need to be kept small. Remember that children's little mouths are much smaller than ours. Use your child's thumbnail or your own little fingernail as a guide to how small pieces should be chopped. Sausages need to be cut lengthwise and then cut lengthwise again before being chopped crosswise into smaller pieces. Grapes need to be halved at the very least. These modifications are to reduce the risk of choking.

Sandwiches are now also a favourite—mainly with mums and dads because they are portable! Start with the crusts off and avoid breads with large grains, fruit pieces or nuts. Quarter the sandwich and then cut the quarters once more as a starting point. Over the 12–15 month period, the chewing muscles will continue to gain strength and efficiency. Children also start to adopt a more efficient grinding or rotary chewing pattern, rather than the infant's munching 'up–down' chewing pattern.

Returning to our walking analogy, now we are starting to learn how to run. Once quartered crustless sandwiches are managed safely and efficiently, try leaving the crusts on. Many parents will say that their children do not eat the crusts and that they end up throwing them out so why leave them on? Leave them on to help develop jaw muscle strength. You need very strong jaw muscles to manage pieces of meat, dried fruit and muesli bars. Adults need about 20 or 30 chewing strokes to safely break down a piece of meat. No wonder children spit out pieces of partly chewed meat. They are still developing those strong chewing muscles, and when the muscles get tired and the tongue sensors detect that the food is unsafe to be swallowed . . . out it comes. You may still end up throwing out some sandwich crusts, but on days when they are very hungry, all of the sandwich will be eaten. A guide to food textures is included in Table 4.

Foods that are a choking risk

Whilst most grown-up foods will now be suitable for your toddler, there are some foods that are best left till your child is about three years old. Extensive research, including research from autopsy studies, has been carried out on the types of food that children most commonly choke on.[3–10] Foods that pose a choking risk have certain textural qualities. These are outlined below. Please note that the examples given provide a guide and are not an exhaustive list. Parents should understand the textural properties of the food and use their judgement to make safe choices for their children.

Table 3: **Foods that pose a choking risk**

Food texture characteristic	Examples	Ways to overcome the choking risk
Stringy Difficult to chew string. The food and string may get lodged part way down the throat.	Rhubarb, beans, celery*	Cut finely, puree or avoid these types of textures until after the age of three.

Food texture characteristic	Examples	Ways to overcome the choking risk
Crunchy Dry-textured and must be chewed well to form small particles.	Popcorn, toast, dry biscuits/crackers,** chips/crisps	Toast should be moistened with a spread and children should be well-supervised at mealtimes. Other crunchy foods are best avoided until after three years of age.
Hard or dry foods These need lots of chewing and grinding down to promote saliva to moisten.	Nuts,* raw broccoli, raw cauliflower, raw carrots, raw apple & apple skin, pork crackling, hard crusted rolls/bread, seeds	Steam or boil broccoli, carrot and cauliflower (stir-frying is not recommended). For under three's: apples should be peeled and sliced into small, paper-thin pieces; breads and rolls should be soft-crusted.
Crumbly Dry foods that need moistening (usually by saliva) to swallow safely.	Dry cakes or biscuits	Choose other foods in preference to these, or provide in small amounts and supervise children well.
Floppy textures Paramedics report that one of the worst things a child could choke on is cellophane because when wet, it sticks to the throat structure above the airway. Floppy textures can do this too.	Lettuce, cucumber, uncooked baby spinach leaves	Alter these food textures by cooking; or with cucumber, present it in chunks to be bitten and chewed rather than as thin rounds.

Food texture characteristic	Examples	Ways to overcome the choking risk
Fibrous or 'tough' Foods with fibre that require a lot of grinding to break down. Jaw muscles need to be strong and well-practised to chew these foods.	Steak, pineapple	Choose soft meats (e.g. chicken, minced meat) and fish. Cut into pieces no larger than your smallest fingernail and ensure child eats only one piece at a time. Finely chop pineapple and similar fibrous foods.
Skins and outer shells These are tougher and more fibrous than flesh, and can get stuck on the lining of the throat.	Corn, peas, unpeeled apple, grapes	Mash peas. Peel apple. Halve or quarter grapes to expose flesh.
Round or long shapes These can block airways.	Whole grapes, whole cherries, raisins, hot dogs, sausages	Cut food into small pieces no larger than your smallest fingernail.
Chewy or sticky These can be difficult to chew down to smaller pieces. Can stick to teeth or roof of mouth. Hard for children to manipulate.	Cheese chunks, fruit roll-ups, gummy lollies, marshmallows, chewing gum, sticky mashed potato, dried fruits	Avoid chewy or sticky foods until child is three years of age. Cut cheese into small pieces and ensure child eats only one piece at a time.
Husks (See earlier in this table under skins and outer shells.)	Corn, bread with grains, shredded wheat, bran	Leave wheat and bran until child is three years of age. Cook corn to soften. Cut grainy breads into small pieces.

Food texture characteristic	Examples	Ways to overcome the choking risk
Mixed consistencies Foods with a liquid and solid in the one mouthful.	Breakfast cereal pieces with milk, minestrone soup, watermelon	Children under three may prefer dry cereal with a cup of milk, rather than mixing together. Ensure a teaspoon is used and each spoonful is swallowed before the next one is attempted. Cut watermelon into fingernail-sized pieces, then gradually increase the size, always ensuring the size is the right proportion for the mouth.

Note: *Denotes foods that are recognised choking risks to children under the age of three years. These foods are best avoided until children are older than three years and have developed adequate chewing skills to safely manage these food textures.

**Biscuits/crackers—These are 'soft' or 'dissolvable' (melt-in-your-mouth) and break down in water within 30 seconds to 1 minute. 'Soft or dissolvable biscuits' will also generally leave crumbs when broken in half. 'Hard' biscuits generally break cleanly into sharp-edged fragments. Biscuits are 'hard' when they have been submerged in water for 2–3 minutes and have not started to dissolve or soften. 'Hard' biscuits are a choking risk for children under the age of three and for children who have not sufficiently developed their chewing strength or stamina.

Brain training—Food textures and flavours

Introducing solid food is also critical for trying new flavours and textures. Each time your child tries a food, they are teaching their brain and their mouth about the food. Let's take a couple of examples. Yoghurt is smooth and the tongue can cup it and control it with little effort. It might take only one or two manipulations and down it goes. A piece of pikelet is soft, but it still needs a bit of chewing before it can be swallowed. What about a hard biscuit? Again chewing is required. But suddenly the brain is figuring out, 'Hey, I need about eight chews for the pikelet but I need about 15 chews for this biscuit'. As we get older, we are well aware of the differences in chewing style required to swallow a marshmallow bolus versus a corn chip bolus. You muck that one up and you end up swallowing sharp spiky bits, which is most uncomfortable! This is the time when we teach our brain about how many chews are required and how much jaw effort is needed for different foods. It is also why we need parental supervision at mealtimes to avoid accidental choking.

Your little one is a novice learner being educated about the wonders of food. So it may take 10–15 presentations of the same food before the child's brain stops saying, 'Hey, that's new! What is that?' Now having said this, we will all have a few foods that we are not fond of for their flavour or texture and that is part of what makes us unique. Julie has vivid memories of her first steak and kidney pie. The flavour was intense and she couldn't stand the texture in her mouth. Neither did she like the feeling of scrambled egg nor meat fat in her mouth; there was a common thread. The slimy lumps that spread throughout her mouth were an intense and unpleasant experience for her. Over time she has learned to manage scrambled eggs, but the others are still firmly off her menu. Just remember, though, that the list of foods we don't like is usually pretty small compared with the foods we will eat, which helps to ensure that we can have a balanced diet. Table 4 below provides an outline of different food textures.

WHAT IF I'VE MISSED A STAGE?

In clinical practice, often some of our younger 'fussy eaters' are little ones who have missed a stage. Mum and Dad may have inadvertently tried to leapfrog some steps and go straight from crawling to running. Chapter 4, 'I've got a "fussy eater", now what do I do?' provides specific techniques for managing when these early phases have been inadvertently missed. There are techniques for helping children who

Table 4: **Food textures**

Texture	Chewing strength required	Examples
Soft and smooth	None	Purees (fruit, vegetable)
Smooth, with soft rounded lumps	Beginner	Mashed, moist foods (e.g. well-mashed or lightly pureed spaghetti bolognese)
Naturally soft foods	Beginner	Banana, avocado
Dissolvable 'hard' solids	Beginner to intermediate	'Melt-in-your-mouth' foods (e.g. wafers, shortbread biscuits, Cruskits)
Hard, dry, non-dissolvable solids	Intermediate to advanced	Baked crackers, some raw fruits and vegetables (e.g. apple, carrot), crunchy muesli bars
Fibrous	Advanced	Red meat, pineapple
Chewy	Advanced	Dried fruit, chewy muesli bars

have missed out on lumpy solids. Similarly, there are strategies for children who are at an age when they are more interested in finger foods than in learning the chewing skills they need for this transition. However, it is important to recognise the problem early and to begin rectifying things as soon as possible. In our experience, time does not help, it hinders. Children do not easily 'grow out of' their feeding issues. Parents need support and guidance to help their children and maintain their own sanity. The next chapter covers one of the most important areas: The age of 'typical food fussiness'. Yes, there is one! It is how we as parents and carers deal with this age that will make all the difference to how our kids come out the other side.

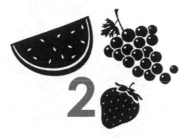

Surviving the age of typical food fussiness
(18 months to three-and-a-half years)

WHAT IS TYPICAL FOOD FUSSINESS AND WHY DOES IT HAPPEN?

The 'terrible twos' are legendary. Parents often describe happy little ones who would eat anything placed in front of them, then one day they woke up and here was this child who refused to eat meals that had previously been eaten with gusto. Anywhere from 18 months to 2½ years your angel may change into a right little devil, and about half of all parents report this phenomenon. It leaves many parents flustered and bewildered because as far as they can see, everything that the parents have done has pretty much remained the same. Here is the critical point. It is *your child* who is changing. Hang in there though, this typical phase generally starts to taper off at around three years of age and continues to gradually reduce over the next couple of years.

BREAST MILK INTRODUCES BABIES TO FOOD FLAVOURS

From the time of conception, babies are being subtly introduced to flavours from Mum's diet. Flavours from the maternal diet are transferred to the amniotic fluid and swallowed by the babies in utero. This flavour journey continues with breastfeeding. Research has shown that flavours from foods eaten by mothers are present in low concentrations in their breast milk.[1] In addition, they have found that flavour intensity in the breast milk peaks at different times for different types of flavours. For example, fruit flavours are barely detectable in breast milk and seem to be present for 1–2 hours at the most after Mum has eaten some fruit. Other flavours, for example, garlic or even carrot juice, have peak flavour concentrations about two hours after consumption.

Researchers have found that there is a great deal of variation in flavour concentration from mother to mother. However, all concentration levels seem to be highly dependent on Mum's diet intake. Researchers are in agreement though that the flavour of breast milk is constantly changing and provides the infant with a cornucopia of subtle flavour variation. Some researchers have even found that mothers who consumed carrot juice during pregnancy and then while breastfeeding had infants who preferred carrot-flavoured cereal to water-based cereals. Infant formula on the other hand provides exactly the same flavour each and every time it is consumed. It may well be that breastfeeding provides the infant with a 'physiological advantage' over formula-fed infants for tolerance of different flavours. This may well have an impact on acceptance of food tastes and flavours during infancy.[2]

GROWTH PATTERNS AND ACTIVITY LEVELS AFFECT EATING BEHAVIOURS

Throughout the first year of life humans grow more rapidly than at any other time (excluding puberty). We often hear grandparents talk about milestones of babies doubling and then quadrupling their birth weight. Indeed many infants have tripled their birth weight by their first birthday. On average, babies in their first three months of life may be gaining about 20–30 g/day.[3] This tapers down to 10–20 g/day by about eight months and then drops to 6–8 g/day from 9–12 months of age. Boys tend to gain more weight than girls. Breastfed babies tend to have slower weight gains than formula-fed infants.

In order for your baby to triple their birth weight in their first 12 months of life, it is no wonder they become a happy little Hoover (vacuum cleaner)! Your baby needs fuel to keep this rapid growth going. Things change considerably, though, on entering the second year of life. Physical growth slows. Let's face it, if we kept growing at the same rate as in our first year of life, we would all end up the size of trees.

In the second year of life the average weight gain per day is about 6 g. Over an entire year this accounts for about 2.4 kg of weight gain.[4] Weight gain each year hovers at about this 2 kg mark until children are around eight years old. Then it gradually creeps up to 3 kg weight gain per year and hits 4 kg per year by ten years of age.[4]

The next big weight gain occurs during puberty, and this time the rapid growth is hormone-driven. For boys we can expect gains of 5 and 6 kg per year through to about 16 years of age, at which stage things taper back down again. Girls have a different growth pattern. From ten to 15 years of age girls will gain a maximum of about 3 to 4½ kg per year, before tapering down again.[4]

Physical activity levels will also play a big part in your child's appetite. A very active toddler will demand more food than the little one happy to sit in the sandpit all day. Many children are notoriously ravenous after a swimming lesson or a big play in the park. Keeping an eye on your child's activity levels will help to provide some clues as to how hungry they might be come mealtimes.

So what does all of this mean to the flustered parent just trying to put meals on the table that their child will eat without too much protest? First of all it means that change in the amount of food your child wants to eat is normal until they stop growing. They generally 'stop growing' when they are ready to leave home! As parents we need to be aware of those peak periods of rapid growth and then be flexible enough to alter *our* expectations of what our child will eat during slower growth periods.

Some parents find it useful to keep track of their child's height and weight using the child health baby book given to many new parents in hospital. This book often holds your child's immunisation details as well. Track your child's height and weight every couple of months and monitor the general pattern over the course of a few months to get a good idea of what is happening. Head circumference is also measured, as growth of the bony skull provides an indication of the brain growing within it. All of these measures are important. Don't become focussed on only your child's weight gain. You will notice that there are different charts for boys and girls. As noted above, this is because boys and girls have different growth patterns. Measuring height and weight is more technical than it sounds. Asking your local doctor or child health nurse to take these measurements can be useful for accuracy. Drops in weight or slowing off of height noted on the charts should be brought to your doctor's attention promptly.

GROWTH SPURTS

Growth spurts sneak up on us and it is often not until the spurt is over that we realise that it has happened. A little head now showing above the kitchen counter where previously goldilocks could be heard but not seen, or pants that are suddenly too small that fitted only two weeks ago, are easily recognised signs of growth spurts. We've noticed with our own children times when they seem especially clumsy, realising later that their legs have grown in length, and a bit like a baby giraffe they can take a little while to adjust to small changes in limb length.

Many babies will go through growth spurts at around seven to ten days after birth, at six to eight weeks of age, and then at three, six and nine months of age. During these times, babies may be extra hungry and seem to be feeding all the time. This pattern often only happens for a few days and then settles again. Often after the feeding frenzy babies may sleep more than usual, and it is thought that this is when the 'growth spurt' per se is happening. Be flexible enough to allow them extra feeds for these days. Because we see our children on a daily basis, we often don't see these small changes happening. It is not until they suddenly seem to grow out of their jumpsuit that you recognise that a growth spurt has occurred.

Toddlers, children and teenagers also go through growth spurts. Similar patterns of increased food intake and being hungry all of the time seem to come, followed by periods of less food intake. Similarly the 'picky or fussy' eating may occur more when there is slow growth happening, with more acceptances of different foods when they are ravenous during fast growth or a 'growth spurt'. While it can make packing a lunchbox a tricky business, this up and down cycle of food intake is perfectly normal and essential to normal growth and development. For parents, this means taking a more flexible approach to expectations of how much and how often children will eat.

News flash! Children have smaller stomachs than older siblings and their parents. Smaller servings are necessary for young children and you can save yourself much angst by providing smaller portion sizes. Children will always ask for more if they are hungry. A bit like the difference in petrol tank size between a Mini Minor and a fire engine, children's tanks empty more quickly than adult tanks. Children need small amounts offered frequently throughout the day. Children obviously need breakfast, lunch and dinner, but also require healthy snacks between meals to keep their little tanks going. So on average, expect to sit your little one down for something to eat about five times a day. A child who has gone a long time between meals is often tired, cranky and ratty. See Chapter 3 for more information on portion size and what constitutes a healthy diet.

Those see-saw periods of bigger appetites around the time of the growth spurt may also gradually increase the size of your child's stomach. It is important to let children eat till they are satisfied and then allow them leave from the table when they have had enough. There is much evidence to show that children are well able to regulate their food intake. If they have a larger or more energy-dense meal, they are often less hungry at the next mealtime.[5] If you encourage your child to listen to their tummy as to when they are hungry and when they are full, you are providing them with valuable information about their body. They can trust their body to know when to eat and when to stop. Problems associated with obesity are likely to be reduced in children who have learned to listen to their body when it comes to eating. Forcing children to eat more than they wish invites a showdown. There is more information for parents in regards to 'mealtime rules' in Chapter 7. The rules are not just for the children, but a code of conduct for parents also.

CHEWING AND SWALLOWING SKILLS—A TIME OF DEVELOPMENT

By about two years of age your child should be well-acquainted with food on the menu at 'Chez My House'. Your earlier efforts at providing one meal for the family from the time of your child's first birthday will have seen them introduced to a wide variety of foods, textures and flavours. Two-year molars will have emerged in all of their glory and your child will have a good set of teeth to attack the amazing world of food. By two of years of age their chewing pattern has very much changed, from an up–down chomping action to a chewing pattern more similar to the one adults use. The 'rotary chewing' pattern allows the back teeth to grind food more efficiently. If you watch closely, you should be able to see that after your child takes a bite of a hard food, they use their tongue to transfer the piece to the side of their mouth and expertly place it between their back teeth for chewing. The food may move from one side of the mouth to the other as the tongue moves the food from left to right. The jaw muscles on both sides of the mouth get a good workout this way. As children get older, they will develop a preferred side where most of their chewing happens. This is normal, in the same way that we have preferences for handedness and even which foot we kick with. It develops with practice and over time.

'Emerging independence: Self-feeding and safe food textures' provided tips on how to improve jaw strength. Parents may mistakenly assume that children will be able to 'just eat' foods with a variety of textures. However, if they have not been exposed to these textures and been able to practise, children will struggle with hard- and fibrous-textured foods. These same foods are, however, essential for providing protein and fibre.

Foods pieces still need to be the right size for little mouths and attempts to overstuff the mouth will likely result in some or all of the food being spat out. Foods that are too tough will also make a reappearance, although your child will often not have the vocabulary to explain exactly why they have spat out that lovely piece of meat. The ability to safely manage hard and fibrous foods takes time and exposure to these foods. A child who has had a very soft diet will struggle and reject hard-textured foods. Be on the lookout for your child clamping their teeth onto a sandwich or a piece of meat and then using all the force their little arms have to rip a piece of food off for chewing. This ripping action often results in a larger mouthful than the child intended and is an indication that the food is too tough for their jaw muscles, hence their compensation with their arms. Similarly, the child who chews and chews and chews and then swallows, or even chews for ages then spits out, may have jaw muscles that are not quite strong enough for that particular food texture.

There may be other reasons why children have difficulty with hard-textured foods. Enlarged or infected tonsils, for example, make it uncomfortable for children to position food on their back teeth for good chewing. These children will have a preference for smooth- and soft-textured foods. They may eat with their mouth open and may also have food left around their mouth after eating. Chapter 5 provides more information about medical and physiological reasons for food fussiness.

A CHANGE IN INDEPENDENCE AND COMMUNICATION

Apart from physical growth over the first two years, there is also a great deal of brain, language and cognitive (thinking) development happening. Even that first smile is a sign of emerging communication. By the time children are one, they will be uttering many one-word sentences: 'Mummy', 'Daddy', 'Billy' and 'Mine'. Imagine also their confusion that the word 'apple' can be applied to a piece of fruit, a drink, a muffin, a cake or a sauce. By their second birthday children are mobile, and often stringing two words together: 'MY Mummy!' They will also have mastered use of the word 'no'. The number of words in a 2-year-old's internal dictionary is way more limited than an adult's. In addition, when asked a question, children often seem to set the default response to 'no'. In regards to food that is offered, 'No' may mean: (a) 'I know what it is and I really don't want it', (b) 'I don't know what it is and "no" is safer than "yes" ', (c) 'I don't want it right now, but I might have it later', (d) 'You laughed and said it was cute last time I said "no" so I'm going for more laughs', or even (e) 'I'm tired and cranky right now and I'm going to say "no" regardless'. Due to developing language skills, children talk in shorthand and we adults provide the interpretation. It's no wonder we have miscommunications! Be aware that children will watch your face to see what kind of response they get. Be careful what face you show them as they often mirror it back to you.

Children's personalities are also developing. Stubborn streaks can become glaringly obvious. These very individual traits will have an impact on your child's temperament. It can often be seen in their decisions of what to put into their mouth and, more importantly for parents, what they will not put into their mouths.

FEEDING SKILLS AND THEIR EFFECT ON SPEECH DEVELOPMENT

Infant feeding skills are closely associated with speech development. The muscles of the lips, face, tongue, soft palate and jaw are all essential for speaking as well as for eating and drinking. Early breastfeeding and bottle-feeding experiences give the tongue, soft palate, lips and jaw muscles a good workout and help these muscle units to work together and get stronger. Your baby learns to groove their tongue to accept the liquid. The tongue is a critical muscle for producing speech sounds. It has to be very strong and very flexible. For example, the tongue tip has an important role with sounds like 't' and 'd', while the back portion of the tongue is essential for sounds like 'k' and 'g'. The tongue has to be fast and flexible to move swiftly from one speech sound to another. Practice with chewing helps the tongue to move around the mouth and become familiar with every nook and cranny.

The lips are important for sounds like 'm', 'p' and 'b'. The soft palate is important for nasal sounds like 'm' and 'n'. During feeding, the soft palate prevents food and liquid from going up into the nose. Later developing sounds like 's' and 'th' need the combined efforts of the lips, tongue and jaw. Like a small acrobatic team, the various muscle groups learn to move seamlessly from one position to the next. Early feeding experiences provide these muscles with a good workout so that they are strong and can hold their positions like little gymnasts during speech. It is common to find that children who have speech disorders have often had feeding difficulties as little ones. It is important to assist your child with any feeding difficulties they may have in order to give them the best start to speech and their way of communicating with the world. A child without clear communication will have their messages misunderstood, leading to frustration and anxiety. Parental intuition is a very good guide for determining when to seek help. If you have concerns regarding your child's communication development, seek the advice of a paediatric speech pathologist.

CAN THERE POSSIBLY BE A 'FEAR' OF NEW FOODS?

So your child has gone from happily opening their mouth like the proverbial baby bird and then one day decides that the jig is up. Suddenly the child that happily ate tuna casserole, chicken and vegetable risotto, and a whole range of fruits and vegetables has been replaced by a child who 'only eats' breakfast wheat biscuits, Vegemite sandwiches, and custard. Not only does the amount of food a child wishes to eat on a daily basis change, but so does their preference for what is on the menu. At about two years of age the variety of what children eat seems to have diminished greatly from what they were eating for their first couple of years.

Interestingly, research has shown that accidental poisonings peak at about the same time as this marked change in eating preferences. Both accidental poisonings and rigidity about food preferences then tail off after this and have usually stabilised by about five years of age.[6] So it may be that, back in the very dim dark ages when apples on trees did not come with stickers or barcodes, nature had a hand in helping little people to learn what things should go into their mouths. Rather than being passive little baby birds, children needed to learn to become independent. They needed to learn for themselves what looked and tasted good, simply to survive till their next birthday.

The foods most rejected by children potentially have the highest risk of toxicity. Many plants cannot be eaten. Many poisons are bitter tasting. If you strike a bitter piece of zucchini, the brain's survival alert mechanisms will trigger most children and many adults to spit out the offending piece of vegetable. Similarly, many animal foods (meat, chicken, fish, milk, egg) can harbour bacteria which can lead to food poisoning. Note also the influence of what a food looks like. It's a bit late to stay alive if you have to put the food in your mouth to confirm that it is poisonous! This may seem far-fetched and extreme; however, the evolution of our species and other species has relied upon us avoiding things that will endanger survival. We need food for fuel. Choosing the wrong fuel is a costly mistake. A hard-wire for food makes for good commonsense. Unfortunately for us, our little Sherlock Holmes is determined to do his or her own experimentation, regardless of our protests.

While there are benefits to this survival mechanism in the form of children spitting out bitter unidentified berries they have found in the garden or Grandma's fish oil tablets, the reality of helping a child through this learning phase is a real test of parental patience. We forget that we are 'experts' in both variety of foods and their various disguises. A 2-year-old may look at you like you've lost your marbles if you show them a whole carrot, a round piece of cooked carrot, a stick of blanched carrot and some grated carrot, and then explain that they are all 'the same'. Clearly you didn't get enough sleep the night before. The whole carrot has bumpy bits on it, is hard and looks good to throw to the dog for fetch. The round of cooked carrot is soft and squishes in my hands. It becomes mushy in my mouth. The blanched carrot stick is harder than the round carrot. I can try my teeth out on it. Sometimes I surprise myself and break off a chunk with my teeth—now what do I do with it? It's too big to swallow in one piece. The grated carrot is wet and sticks to my hands. If I put a handful in my mouth suddenly there are lots of little bits in my mouth for me to control with my tongue so I don't choke. What did you call this again? All of it 'carrot'? The next time you offer me 'carrot' I'm not quite sure what will end up on my plate. Return to the safety of the default setting—the answer is 'NO!'

An average 30-year-old adult will have eaten about 27,000 meals (giving leeway for their own period of food fussiness between ages 2 and 5 years!). In addition, you may also have consumed about 20,000 snacks over this time. You know what all the different vegetables, fruits, meats, breads, cakes, chocolates, cheese, etc. look like and taste like. You are an expert. You are not fazed if someone hands you a casserole because you readily identify the chunks of meat, the cubes of potato, the chunks of carrots, broccoli and tomato. You know that just because a carrot and a potato touch each other, they do not become a 'potatocarrot' with new taste properties. You understand that when you put a spoonful of casserole into your mouth there will be hard chunks, smooth chunks and a sauce. That's three different textures to deal with in your mouth. Your child is a novice. They have none of these skills. They acquire these skills by gradual and patient introductions by a loving and understanding coach over many years. Welcome to the job, coach!

Someone once said that we take our first 'bite' of food with our eyes. The way a food looks certainly has an impact on our likelihood of putting it anywhere near our mouth. If you've travelled by plane, you will appreciate the apprehension with which you lift the lid on your little foil pack to look at its contents. The facial expressions of the adults as well as the children can be pretty spectacular. So now imagine yourself in a new country. You have just been provided with a dish the likes of which you have never seen before. You gingerly pick up a fork and prod the food to get an idea of whether it is firm or soft. You might separate bits of the meal to see how they differ. Feeling very brave, you might take a portion on your fork and bring it up towards your mouth. Bringing it close to your mouth allows the aroma to waft up your nose. You bring the fork to your mouth where the fine sensory receptors on your lips will feel the food, giving your brain the first glimpse of what to expect once the food is in your mouth. Your tongue touches the food and more intense sensations occur, together with flavour. At this point you may try a small bite. If the piece is particularly chewy or does not feel pleasant in the mouth or the flavour too overpowering or spicy, we will find a way to politely remove the offending morsel. So why is it then that we tell children not to poke or play with their food, to 'just take a mouthful and eat it' and then get cross with them when they make faces and spit it out? This 'trying a new food' thing has quite a few steps to it. We need to be sympathetic to those steps and teach our children *how* to try a new food.

It takes 10–15 presentations of the same food or drink before we become accustomed to the taste, aroma, mouth-feel and texture of a food. Those 10–15 presentations do not all happen in one sitting, mind you! It is a gradual and deliberate process. It is as though the brain is saying 'Hey that's new', and with each new presentation working out a way to categorise the food. It can take the better part of a month or more, with small but consistent offerings of the same food, before the child accepts a particular food. Unfortunately, many parents stop after the third presentation. We need to be positive and persistent, particularly with foods that are essential to growth, health and wellbeing.

CHILDREN'S FOOD PREFERENCES FROM TWO TO THREE YEARS OF AGE

As you might imagine, designing studies to look objectively at what children choose to eat away from their parents' guiding hands is rare. Well-designed studies to look at children's eating patterns are also difficult to come by. There have been a few good studies where children's food choices and eating patterns have been observed. In one study, children who attended a crèche were observed. Children were able to self-serve from a selection of foods from the categories offered: animal products (meats, fish, chicken and egg), dairy products (yoghurt, cheese and milk), starchy foods (bread, pasta and rice), and vegetables and fruits. No dessert items were offered. Children took a serving spoon of whatever they wished and returned to their table to eat. They were able to choose more food if they had finished what they had chosen.

Almost all children chose animal products or starchy foods (French fries, pasta, mashed potato, sausage, breaded fish, roast beef and chicken). The choice of dairy products depended on the type of food on offer, with yoghurt and cream cheese being more frequently chosen than mature cheese, for example. The 'dairy food group' was the only whole food group completely avoided by a small percentage of the children (7 per cent). Vegetables were generally the last thing chosen, if chosen at all (think cabbage, cauliflower, salad and lettuce). Interestingly, vegetables in a sauce were more acceptable than vegetables on their own.

A DIET DICTATED BY FOOD TEXTURE

Some children's diets change because of their textural preferences for the food they eat. Unfortunately, variety is the biggest issue with these profiles. Children who show a preference for soft foods may need to develop their strength and stamina for chewing skills. These children are missing valuable fibre and possibly also iron due to reduced protein intake through lack of red meat in their diet. Children who prefer dry foods may lack calcium and also have a general reduction in food variety, which limits their nutritional balance. Children who prefer 'white foods' also have severely restricted food variety that reduces the range of textures they will tolerate. Some children seek out dry, soft, white foods. More than any other, this group needs help to develop chewing skills and guidance to experience new food textures and tastes to allow variety. Children in this group may suffer problems associated with deficiencies of calcium, iron, vitamin C and potassium. They may be irritable, show short attention spans and suffer from constipation.

Similarly, children's flavour choices may help a parent to tailor their child's snacks. Children who enjoy the taste of Vegemite, salami and tomato paste may have a more savoury palate. Some parents have commented that their child has a 'sweet tooth' because they enjoy chocolate. However, some children enjoy the taste of chocolate, but reject lollies and other confectionery. Chocolate has bitter qualities, and so cannot be used to indicate that a child 'only likes' sweet foods. If the enjoyment of chocolate occurs alongside a hearty appetite for sweet biscuits, cakes and other confectionery, then it is likely that a preference for sweet foods can be attributed. Some common profiles are shown in the table below.

Table 5: Diet according to food texture and flavour preferences resulting in nutritional inadequacies

General description of preferred foods	Child *prefers* to eat	Child *avoids* eating
Dry foods	Sandwiches, biscuits, chicken nuggets, chicken chippies, pomme potatoes, fish fingers, sometimes apple, sometimes corn on the cob	Meat (beef, lamb, pork), mashed potatoes, fruit, vegetables in all forms, rice, couscous
Soft foods	Milk, yoghurt, banana, mandarin, cooked rolled oats (porridge), Weetbix with milk, cheese slice, sausage, hot potato chips, potato crisps, custard, wafers, fruit puree, ice-cream, tinned spaghetti, two-minute noodles, doughnuts, chicken nuggets, fish fingers, sultanas, sandwiches (crusts removed), bolognaise sauce	Raw vegetables, meat (all types except sausages), fruit, bran cereal, pizza

General description of preferred foods	Child *prefers* to eat	Child *avoids* eating
White foods	Sandwiches (crusts removed), milk, yoghurt, plain pasta, custard, plain biscuits (e.g. Arrowroot), chicken nuggets, fish fingers, chocolate, bagels, croissants	Red meat, bolognaise sauce, fruit, vegetables, mashed potatoes, bran cereal, couscous, pizza
Savoury foods	Plain, savoury or salt and vinegar potato crisps, hot potato chips, salad dressing, tzatziki dip, sour light cream, chocolate, toast, plain breakfast cereal (e.g. Cornflakes, Rice Bubbles), yoghurt (lemon or vanilla flavour), sultanas, bolognaise sauce, garlic bread, chapati, pizza, baked beans	Fruit, overly sweet cakes and biscuits, gummy lollies
Sweet foods	Chocolate, sweet cakes and biscuits, sweet breakfast cereal, ice-cream, ice blocks, fruit (most!), bolognaise sauce, English muffin, toast, pizza	Vegetables, meat, fish, savoury dips, savoury potato crisps, bran cereal, rice paper wrappers (e.g. used on spring rolls)

Sauces can be used as a flavour bridge to help a child accept a new food. BUT, do not be tempted to mix vegetables together. The vegetable hotpot is far less likely to be chosen than if the vegies were presented in their own little piles so that carrots don't get 'potato germs' and vice versa. Keeping foods separate in the early stages helps children to learn to recognise these foods in their different disguises, like the carrots referred to earlier. However, once children are around 3½–4 years or older, it is important to show them that foods can be happily placed and eaten together.

We know that intake of fruit and vegetables is important. Many parents will describe that their child will eat a reasonable variety of fruits but struggles with the vegetables. Fruits may be better tolerated because of their sweetness. Human breast milk is sweet, and it appears we are physiologically pre-programmed to seek sweet-tasting foods.[7] Vegetables are not naturally sweet, and are often fibrous. However, vegetables are essential for their vitamin and mineral content. While they provide very little by way of kilojoules or calories, their nutrients and fibre react with other foods to enhance growth and repair our systems. So even though we know they are good for us, why do we struggle so much to eat our quota of five veggies every day?

As an analogy, think back to the old Pac-Man computer games. Pac-Man would go around the screen and gobble up round circles. Each circle eaten gave Pac-Man 1 point. Sometimes Pac-Man would come across a different-coloured circle and this special circle would give a bonus 20 points. Foods can be similar to the circles in the Pac-Man game. Our fruits and vegetables are like the ordinary 1-point circles in the Pac-Man game and they are important to keep us going. On the other hand, protein foods (e.g. meat, dairy) are like the special different-coloured circles. In the computer game, Pac-Man has to eat lots of the ordinary circles and there are only a few special circles to be eaten. However, outside the computer-game world, changes in our lifestyle have made it such that the 'special circles' are far more freely available to humans. So if you were Pac-Man, and suddenly there were lots of 'special circles' available to you, what would you prefer? Lots of the 'ordinary circles'? Or lots of the 'special circles'? Children are not silly. They don't need adults to tell them the answer. Their body has been designed over the centuries to work it out for them. Given a choice, children will happily eat foods that provide them with kilojoules for growing and shy away from the foods that are still important but have less palatable flavour and texture than higher kilojoule foods.

Here's a scary thought. Many commercially available, processed and 'ready-to-go' foods are specially designed to be easy to eat, high in energy and especially nice to taste. Think about how long it takes you to eat a fast food hamburger as opposed to a piece of steak, salad and a bread roll. The actual amount of these fast foods we need to eat is small because they are packed with kilojoules. The downside is that there is little fibre, excessive sugar, fat and salt, and many colours, flavours and additives to make it 'taste good'.

WHAT DRIVES THEIR FOOD PREFERENCES?

At around two years of age children are becoming more in tune with their bodies and learning to recognise what they do and don't like, and this includes the flavour and textures of food. After some initial experimentation, children will decide what their favourites are and cling to them like a safety net. This behaviour does not just occur with food, however. Most families will have dog-eared copies of a few children's books because these favourites were read multiple times daily, for weeks on end. Many parents can still recite some books by heart even years after their last intensive reading session! Think also of those coloured-skivvy clad fellows and their big red car. Many of these DVDs wear out from being played over and over again between those magic ages of two and three years. So, really, food just follows this natural progression. 'I like it like this! I like it like this all the time! Be very brave if you're going to try to change my mind!' And then just as quickly as a fad started, it changes to a new one, and then ever so gradually it disappears.

As adults, we still have traces of the 'I like it like this "gene" ' too. Many adults have a favourite dish at a favourite restaurant. There is that hunger in anticipation of the first mouthwatering morsel because they know what to expect and just how much they enjoy it. It can be a very deliberate step for adults to choose a new menu item. We have all at times been disappointed if the new dish doesn't live up to our enjoyment of our old-favourite menu offerings. Sticking to what we know can often be safer.

As noted above, there will be some foods that are universal favourites and some that are universal cast-asides. The rest will develop based on your own little cosmos and picket-fence experiences. Children will also choose because of the way the food feels on their lips and tongue or in their mouth. Avoidance of fibrous textures (apples, celery, cabbage) is an indicator that the child has not developed the chewing skills or stamina for these foods. If these foods are not chewed properly, they are a choking risk. The child's brain is very clever. Poorly chewed fibrous foods will be spat out rather than risk choking. The way a food tastes will also affect food acceptance. Foods that are bitter (e.g. brussel sprouts) or sour (e.g. tomato) may be rejected. Always be aware, though, that we often default to taste as the culprit, when sometimes food texture may be the real problem. Julie's youngest can tolerate the taste of strawberries, but strongly dislikes the 'nuts'. When Kate asked him to show her these 'nuts', he said 'They are everywhere', calmly pointing to the seeds on the outside of the strawberry. Sometimes taste and texture can combine for a diabolical combination. Even though a food may be high in energy density and a 'desirable' food because you get more energy from it, the sensation of the food in your mouth can put you right off.

Some children will cope with foods cooked or presented in one format and completely reject them in another format. For example, cucumbers may be better tolerated if peeled and the seeds are removed initially. Grape tomatoes are less acidic than cherry tomatoes. You might even try removing the tomato seeds on first tries. Using a vegetable peeler you can peel strips of carrot or cucumber and provide these thin ribbons for 2½-year-olds and older children to try. A number of children prefer this style of raw vegetable to cooked vegetables. If you find a format that your child enjoys their fruit or veggies in, stick with it during this phase and gently introduce alternatives over time.

HOW THE WHEELS FALL OFF AND THE 'FUSSY EATER' IS BORN

Let's put all of these events together, look into the crystal ball and see what begins to emerge. We have a child who is naturally starting to slow down the incredible food intake that their parents have become accustomed to over their first 18 months of life. They are naturally starting to eat less. Although growth has slowed, they continue to have growth spurts which see periodic increases in appetite. However, trying to predict when these food increases will happen is a bit like trying to pick lottery numbers. During their slow growth periods children are enjoying foods that they 'adore', much like their beloved bedtime story, TV program or movie. Boring sure, but safe and dependable. They know exactly what to expect of these foods. During their faster growth periods they may be more adventurous with food and willing to try something a little different. This will usually happen when you are visiting Great Aunt Hilda and have just explained that there is no way that Charlie will even touch an olive, let alone allow one to pass his tender lips. He will then, on cue, devour most of the platter.

We also have a child who is starting to look intensely at the environment and carefully and systematically explore that environment for themselves. Fortunately, they are now far less likely to be found eating from the dog's bowl. Rather than being passive eating machines, they are now careful connoisseurs of what goes into their mouth. Evolution has played its part and children are now wary of dog food, unusual plants and most items placed on their dinner plates. In days gone by, this food neophobia was critical to ensure survival of the species. Now parents just want to survive the 'neophobic toddler species'!

Add to all of this a little person who is learning how to communicate. Like a Morse code machine, children have only learned the basics of sending and receiving messages. Parents are learning how to decode their little cherubs and many miscommunications are bound to occur. Patience, patience and more patience is required of tired parents. It is little wonder that most family feuds occur at dinnertime, when everyone in the household is tired.

Trying to make sense of all of these changes, parents tend to go with what their child will eat. If they have suddenly stopped eating chicken risotto, but are eating chicken nuggets, well, they're still getting some protein, aren't they? Concerned that their little one will starve if they don't eat dinner one night, some families will tear the kitchen apart to create a dinner that the child will eat. Having found a 'dinner winner', and preferring not to go through such turmoil again, the same few dinners become regular mealtime features. It is highly unlikely that these few dinners will consist of fruit and vegetables.

Evolution has also had a part here, and meals are more likely to consist of some variety of dairy (custard, milk, yoghurt), protein (chicken, fish, minced meat) and carbohydrates (bread, pasta).[8] With luck there may also be some fruit, but vegetables may be viewed with abject horror. Attempts to introduce something new will be met with the default setting response of 'NO'. Like trying to entice a person with a fear of heights to bungy-jump, many parental attempts to have their child try new foods are futile. Parents throw their hands up in despair and the 'fussy eater' is born.

Problems then become firmly entrenched when parents refer to their child as a 'fussy eater' and tell children that they 'do not like' vegetables or fruit or whatever else may be on offer. If you play the same message over enough times, your listener will believe you. Certainly there is an art to introducing new foods which makes good sense once you are aware of it. So, if you already have a fussy eater, read on for some tips to help bring back peace of mind and smooth mealtimes. Research confirms that the first four years of life are essential for establishing your child's food repertoire.[9] All of the hard work is worth the effort in the long-term.

ADVICE TO PARENTS

- Food fussiness is a typical developmental phase that occurs with children around the age of two to three years of age (but sometimes as early as 18 months). Forewarned is forearmed!

- Accept that the variety of foods your child will eat may well decline during this period of time. Continue to offer new foods, but accept that old favourites will be demanded.

- The way you handle your responses during this time will, to a large extent, determine how you and your child come out the other end. Remain calm, positive and provides lots of encouragement for any attempts to touch, smell, lick, taste or bite a new food. Reward your child for 'trying' and they will be more inclined to continue to try new foods. 'Trying' does NOT mean eating a whole piece or even a whole bite.

- Continue to prepare one meal for the family. Include one item from the 'demanded' list, but keep the remainder as you would for the rest of the family, making adjustments with cutting food to smaller size for smaller mouths, etc.

- The most favourable window for introducing a wide variety of different tastes and textures occurs within the first two years of life. However, there are benefits to continuing to offer new foods many times over to expose children to different food tastes and textures. Children need to be taught *how* to try new foods, and parents need to be patient while children are learning. The food choices we make in the first few years will have a long-term effect, following your child through their childhood, adolescence and into adulthood.

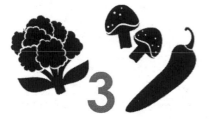

What is a good diet?

'I am just so frustrated. He used to be such a good eater until he turned two. Now all he eats is plain pasta, rice crackers and milk! I'm really worried. Is this going to cause any long-term nutritional problems or damage his health?'

This scenario is common in any family who has a child less than five years of age. Children are strange little creatures who thrive on routine and yet cause angst amongst parents and carers by changing their minds almost daily when it comes to what they are prepared to eat. One day they are happy to wolf down a bowl of spaghetti bolognaise only to turn their nose up at it when offered again a few days later. The main concern for parents is the nutritional adequacy of their little one's diet. If they are fussy and avoiding whole groups of foods, how will that affect the growth and development of their child?

The first consideration when it comes to addressing children's feeding issues is looking at their diet as a whole and comparing it to a 'good diet' which provides all the necessary nutrients required for growth at varying ages. If parents keep a record of exactly what their child eats for a few days and compare it favourably to a reference diet, then the issue can become a lot less worrying for everyone concerned.

THE BARE ESSENTIALS—WHAT CONSTITUTES A GOOD DIET?

A 'good diet' consists of an amount of food required from each food group to satisfy the child's daily recommended dietary needs.

Our food supply is broken into five groups:

1. Fruits
2. Vegetables
3. Dairy (including goat's milk and soy products)
4. Breads, cereals and grains
5. Protein (including red meat, chicken and pork), eggs, fish, legumes and nuts.

Fruits and vegetables

It is common knowledge that fruits and vegetables are important as essential building blocks of any diet. Not only are they loaded with vitamins and minerals which are essential for healthy living, but they also help fill you up, as part of a balanced diet. They provide a great source of fibre which is extremely important in maintaining a healthy gut. They also help to avoid constipation, a common complaint suffered by children (see also Chapter 5). Increasing the intake of fruit and vegetables will help to boost the immune system, as well as build resistance to common illnesses and infections. We should consume two serves of fruit and five serves of vegetables every day. This may sound initially like a large proportion of your child's daily overall intake, but it is essential that we strive to meet this target for the benefit of your child's physical and mental health.

Fruit is a great substitute for sugary snacks, which otherwise deplete energy and lead to numerous other health problems including tooth decay, tiredness and irritability in children, something we could all do without! The natural sugar contained within fruits, known as fructose, is absorbed more slowly than foods containing sucrose. Therefore fruits provide slow release, long lasting energy. Highly processed and refined foods in children's diets today are being blamed as one of the major contributing factors towards our obesity epidemic. Vegetables should account for a substantial proportion of each meal, providing a large amount of fibre and also essential vitamins, minerals and antioxidants.

Dairy (including calcium-fortified soy products)

Dairy foods such as milk, cheese, custard and yoghurt are a critical part of every child's diet as it is these foods that are the major contributor of dietary calcium. Calcium is an essential nutrient involved in the healthy growth of bones, teeth, nails and muscles. Dairy foods are a leading source of many other essential nutrients including protein, phosphorus, potassium, riboflavin, vitamin A, vitamin B12, niacin and vitamin D (if fortified). Because milk and other dairy products are calcium-rich, nutrient-dense foods, their intake improves the overall nutritional quality of children's diets.

Breads, cereals and grains

Breads, cereals and grains make up the largest part of children's diets. They provide a good source of slow release carbohydrates and fibre. Foods that are good sources of fibre are beneficial because they're filling and, therefore, discourage overeating. Pleasantly, fibre itself adds no kilojoules. Plus, when combined with drinking adequate fluids, eating high-fibre breads and cereals helps to move food through the digestive system and protect against gut cancers and constipation. It may also lower cholesterol as well as help prevent diabetes and heart disease in adulthood.

Protein

Many foods contain small amounts of protein but the best sources are beef, poultry, fish, eggs, dairy products, nuts, seeds, and legumes like chickpeas, lentils and soybeans. Protein is another essential nutrient for children especially in the fast growing phases of early childhood. It builds up, maintains and repairs tissues in the body. Muscles, organs and the immune system are made up mostly of protein. Protein foods have another important role to play in children's diets in helping to keep children satisfied. Protein in the meal helps to delay the emptying of the stomach, therefore making them feel fuller for longer. Protein also helps to slow the release of sugars into our bloodstream, therefore giving us a more sustained energy. This is of great benefit to both children and parents in limiting the little power surges followed by energy slumps often seen multiple times in a child's day.

FOOD PORTIONS—HOW MUCH AT EACH AGE?

Children need to eat a variety of nutritious foods, in the right proportions. They should also eat items from each of the five food groups on a daily basis, unless they have a food allergy (see Chapter 5). Foods high in saturated fats or sugar should be eaten only occasionally and in small amounts—think about those birthday parties where after a session at the party table we often see complete personality changes in our little angels! Variations in serving sizes reflect children's different body sizes and activity levels. The main liquids recommended for children are water and milk. Children over the age of two should consume reduced-fat milk and be encouraged to drink water when they are thirsty. Fruit juice is not recommended as an alternative to water, and soft drinks should be avoided.

In the following table you will find an approximate guide to the number of serves children aged one to five years require of each of the different food groups.

Table 6: **Approximate daily needs for children one to five years of age**

Food group	One year	Two years	Three years	Four years	Five years	What is one 'serve'?
Breads and cereals	4 serves	4 serves	5 serves	5 serves	5 serves	1 slice bread ½ bread roll 2 plain biscuits ½ to 1 cup of cereal ½ cup of porridge 1 cereal biscuit ½ cup cooked pasta ½ cup cooked rice
Fruits and vegetables	3 serves	4 serves	4 serves	4 serves	4 serves	1 piece fruit ¼ cup vegetables ½ potato ½ carrot
Dairy	3 serves	3 serves	3 serves	3 serves	3 serves	200 ml milk 200 ml yoghurt 200 ml custard 40 g cheese
Meat and alternatives	1 serve	2 serves	2 serves	2 serves	2 serves	30 g meat, fish or poultry 1 egg 1 tablespoon peanut paste 2 tablespoons hommus ½ cup baked beans 1 fish finger
Fats and oils	1 serve	1 serve	2 serves	2 serves	2 serves	2 teaspoons

The great thing about having foods categorised into groups is that we can balance the diet using other foods from the same group. If a child decides that red meat is off the menu for the time being, then we can substitute chicken, fish, eggs or legumes to provide the protein, zinc and iron that would have otherwise come from red meat. The key is balance and knowing when and what to substitute when individual foods or whole groups of foods are in a 'Mexican stand-off' with your child.

You should not base your child's diet on one individual day. It is better to look at a whole week to assess the nutritional adequacy of their diet. It is not uncommon for children to eat erratically. We see this in adults at Christmas time. We go from one group of grandparents to another and possibly catch up with friends. At each of these places we eat (to be polite of course!), but the effect is that we end up overeating for the day. Over the next couple of days our body compensates and we generally eat less. Children seem to adopt the 'Christmas day eating cycle' every week. One day it may seem as though they may consume enough for two children whereas the following day they seem to exist solely on the air they breathe. Children, unlike most adults, know when they are hungry and are great at regulating their appetite. They also know when they are full. We need to listen to this if they are going to grow up having a healthy relationship with food.

In the following table you will find some example menu plans for children of varying ages. These menu plans have been devised to provide a balanced diet with all essential food groups, minerals, micronutrients and macronutrients.

Table 7: Menu plan examples for children of varying ages

Age group	Menu plan
1–3-year-olds	5 glasses of water **Breakfast** ½ cup iron-fortified cereal + milk (full cream for under twos) 80–100 g yoghurt **Morning tea** Crackers and hommus Sultanas **Lunch** Vegemite and cheese (full cream for under twos) sandwich (wholegrain bread) **Afternoon tea** Banana Carrot (blanched), cucumber and cream cheese **Dinner** Salmon rissoles (with 40–60 g salmon) and vegetables
4–8-year-olds	6 glasses of water **Breakfast** ¾ cup iron-fortified cereal + reduced-fat milk 150 ml milk **Morning tea** Yoghurt (reduced-fat) and grapes **Lunch** Tuna, tomato and cream cheese pita bread Carrot sticks **Afternoon tea** Apple Wholegrain crackers and peanut paste **Dinner** Mexican burritos (with 80 g meat, lettuce, tomato and cheese)

Age group	Menu plan
9–13-year-olds	8 glasses of water **Breakfast** 1+ cup iron–fortified cereal + reduced-fat milk Toast and egg or baked beans **Morning tea** Fruit and yoghurt **Lunch** Chicken, salad and avocado roll Reduced-fat flavoured milk **Afternoon tea** Cheese and crackers Dried fruit **Dinner** 100 g meat, lamb chops and 1 cup vegetables
14–18-year-olds	9 glasses water **Breakfast** Iron-fortified cereal + reduced–fat milk Toast + spreads Fruit smoothie (reduced-fat milk) **Morning tea** Crackers + hommus Strawberries Yoghurt drink **Lunch** 1–2 egg and lettuce sandwiches (multigrain bread) Mandarin **Afternoon tea** Vegetable sticks with avocado and cream cheese dip Reduced–fat flavoured milk **Dinner** 100–150 g chicken, chicken kebabs with peanut satay sauce and 2 cups of vegetables

WHAT TO DO WHEN IMPORTANT FOODS ARE AVOIDED

To us the term 'food fights' conjured up pictures of teenage girls and boys at school camps tossing food at one another until the teacher in charge or 'sergeant major' entered the hall and demanded some order. Nowadays the age of the child is younger, there is a little tossing of food, usually on the floor, and the parent is the one who feels they have lost all control. Parents feel under the complete control of the defiant little 'sergeant major' in the chair. Many parents report the feeling of dinnertime warfare night after night, which is no fun for anyone in the home. As discussed earlier the first line of defence is nutritional balance. The key is finding at least one food in every group that your child likes or will eat.

Fussy fruit bats

If they like pears and bananas but flatly refuse to even try strawberries, apples, pineapple or any other fruit that you put in front of them, this is fine in the interim. Children usually like routine and repetition and many are happy to have an apple every morning tea for a year. As they get older you will find that their palates mature and they are happy to try new things. Do you like every fruit offered to you? Rockmelon, Kate admits, is not in her top 100!

Fruit can be prepared in different ways, such as threaded on small skewers, chopped into little pieces, mixed with sultanas, or cooked into foods such as banana pikelets, apple muffins or mango smoothies. What you are trying to do is introduce a new taste that is made more subtle using familiar foods. Having other 'super eaters' around your child to share in the experience will often encourage them to try something new. Cutting fruit into small bite-size pieces is visibly less daunting to consume than a whole fruit. Chilling fruits or blending and freezing with low-fat yoghurt and placing in an ice-cream cone is a sure-fire way of making them lick it and at least taste it. Recent research has suggested that children may need to be offered a new food at least ten times before they are even willing to touch it, let alone try it.

Dried fruit is a good substitute for fresh fruit, however, these do lack the vitamin C levels contained in the fresh ones. Avocado is also classified as a fruit, so if they enjoy using avocado as a dip mixed with cream cheese, ricotta cheese or plain yoghurt, then you have found a great substitute. Don't be afraid to try different combinations of foods—Kate believes banana and avocado mixed together is a taste sensation!

The 'non-vegetable embracers'

Vegetables are one of the most difficult food groups to get a child to try, let alone enjoy. They are usually the last food to be left on the dinner plate and so have often gone cold. Cold plain vegetables left to the end of the meal will often reduce an otherwise happy child to floods of tears with intermittent bouts of dry retching whilst they are being forced to sit at the table until they are finished. It is a lot easier to mix vegetables, with their strong distinctive tastes, into main meals such as frittatas, quiches, sauces (including bolognaise and cheese sauces), meatloaves, patties and rissoles. Then you know that your child is getting the vitamins, minerals and fibre in their meal. Vegetables do change the taste of the meals so children's palates get used to less bland tastes and they eventually recognise the different vegetable tastes. Kate is a fan of cooking vegetables and blending them to be used as a spread on pizza bases, sandwiches or mixed with yoghurt as a dip. Again you will feel confident knowing they are getting vitamins, minerals, antioxidants and fibre without the hassle of having them avoid the vegetables in their whole form. It is easier to negotiate with an older child the benefits of vegetables and health. Hiding vegetables is not a new concept; however, hiding them in chocolate cakes and sweets is, and we must admit we don't agree with this practice (see Chapter 6).

Dairy avoidance or obsession!

It is unusual for children to avoid all dairy products. The more common problem is milk avoidance whilst consuming cheese and yoghurt, or consuming no other dairy than milk. Probably one of the most common fussy eating problems Kate sees is children addicted to milk, whilst consuming very little of anything else. Milk for many children does become an addiction, especially if solids are not introduced appropriately or bottles are used for too long. Exasperated parents have also used the milk option when all meals have been rejected. 'She simply would not eat any dinner so we gave her a bottle of milk to fill her up before bed and so she wouldn't be hungry.' This is an easy trap to fall into and a hard one to climb out of.

The key with dairy is to ensure three serves of calcium-rich dairy or soy. This can be in the form of milk, yoghurt or cheese. Make sure you buy calcium-enriched soy milk. Cheese is a very versatile calcium- and protein-rich food and can be added to many dishes. For example, sprinkling it over the top as on pizza, cooking into the meal such as in quiches, making a white cheese sauce, baking into muffins and scrolls, or using it in a creamed form as a dip or spread. Yoghurt is also versatile as it can be used as a sweet on its own or with fruit. Yoghurts can be frozen with fruit to make an 'ice-cream alternative'. In addition, it can also be used in its natural plain form as a sauce or dip or mixed with vegetables and meat to make a paste.

If you feel your child is relying too heavily on milk, it may be time to assess the dietary practices. A cup should have replaced the bottle by the first birthday. Try to encourage a serve of cheese each day as well as a serve of yoghurt, which contains beneficial probiotics, or good bacteria, to maintain a healthy gut. Then you are left with one serve of dairy or calcium-enriched soy to balance the day. Many parents find when they reduce the amount of milk that their child consumes (against the child's 'better judgement') that they have a surge in appetite and interest in trying new foods.

It is worth noting that when a 'major' change is to be implemented in a child's diet—such as changing bottles to cups, getting rid of dummies or not cooking chicken nuggets as a separate meal—all parties involved in the care of the child (including daycare, grandparents and friends) are united, otherwise it will not work. Inconsistencies just encourage the child to develop a stronger will as they learn that if they are defiant enough someone will give in.

Breads, cereals and wholegrains—Don't like the chewy bits

There is a common group of children known as the 'white food' consumers. They like everything white, from white bread to pasta to rice crackers to milk. They are not fond of sauces or anything mixed with these white foods (see also Chapter 4). These foods by themselves are very bland and low in protein, iron, fibre, vitamins and minerals. However, they are extremely easy to eat and don't involve a lot of chewing. Some children don't have much jaw strength or chewing stamina, which also contributes to the problem. It is important to try to substitute white foods with a few wholegrain crackers and wholemeal or wholegrain bread, to increase the fibre and value of wholegrains in the diet.

Cereals are a power pack of energy and nutrients and can be eaten at breakfast or eaten dry as a snack. Look for cereals that are fortified with iron and have fibre. If your child won't eat them with milk, don't worry. They will probably have a glass of milk or a tub of yoghurt later. Eating foods on their own and not combining foods is also common and children will eventually realise that foods complement each other. A great cereal, which is commonly overlooked in children over 12 months of age, is the baby rice cereal. It is fortified with iron and has a small amount of protein so it can be added to things like sauces and baked goods such as scones, pikelets, pancakes or yoghurt, especially if they are avoiding cereal.

The non-meat eater

This is by far the most common food avoidance in children under the age of five. Avoiding this group is also the one that holds the highest risk for deficiencies, namely iron and zinc deficiency. These deficiencies are becoming more and more common in the developing world. Iron is involved in the transport of oxygen around the body and is an integral part of running the immune system. Zinc is a major player in healthy skin and the reproductive organs. Iron and zinc are two of the most important nutrients in a child's diet. If the diet is lacking in these elements, it may be necessary to supplement under medical supervision. Before such measures are taken, it is helpful to know that iron occurs in many other foods, such as legumes and tofu. You can spread hommus (blended chickpeas) on pizza bases or sandwiches or use as a sauce or dip, and it is a great meat substitute. Lentils can be added to pastas and soups (red lentils almost dissolve so they can't be detected!) as a meat alternative. Silken tofu can also be added to frittatas or anything with a pouring sauce.

As already suggested, baby rice cereal can top up the iron in the diet. Iron-fortified cereals are also a necessity in the diet of young children. Take them to the supermarket and let them select from a few you choose. We are often asked about the 'cereals that are high in sugar'. A good guide for picking cereal is to choose one with wholegrains, that is iron-fortified and with less than around 1 teaspoon or 5 g of sugar per serve. Remember if you choose one that has little or no sugar and add a tablespoon of honey—you will end up with 16–18 g of sugar anyway!

An egg is another miracle food. We often refer to it as nature's little vitamin capsule. Boiled, scrambled, poached or made into French toast, eggs are a great meat alternative. Eggs can also be included in baking or made into baked custards or sauces. Be careful with raw eggs and smoothies as it is not recommended to give raw eggs to children due to the risk of salmonella poisoning.

Zinc is found in many of the same foods as iron but by far the greatest source is fish and seafood. White fish has a very bland flavour and soft texture and children usually love it. We have seen a decrease in the consumption of fish and seafood over the past ten years, as many families don't like preparing it or only consume it as fish and chips. Therefore it has become an 'only once a week or fortnight' food. We need to increase the consumption of fish and seafood, considering its nutritional benefits. Try pasta bakes, rissoles and patties, fish balls, or dry-fried or barbecued, crumbed fish. Prawns and lightly fried calamari can also be a hit.

I've got a 'fussy eater', now what do I do?

It doesn't seem to matter who you talk to, in most families, there is at least one 'fussy eater'. The term 'fussy eater' is routinely used regardless of whether the little cherub is six months, 16 months, or 16 years of age! And as adults, our ideas of 'fussy' can be as different as the number of colours in a jar of hundreds and thousands. Some of the patterns that children adopt are associated with their age or stage of development. So, if you've jumped straight to this chapter, it is worth your while to read Chapters 2 and 3 as well. Some children, however, seem to be 'sent to test us'.

First and foremost, please do not refer to your child as a 'fussy eater' anywhere in their hearing range. Hearing the same message over and over causes that thinking to become ingrained. 'He's such a fussy eater' becomes 'It's my job in this family to be the fussy eater'. Some children are proud to be non-fruit consumers! For older children, food may be the first thing their parents talk about when they are dropped over to a friend's to play: 'Oh, don't worry if she doesn't eat much—she's such a fussy eater.' Now even if there is something the child might have actually tried there, they are going to be less likely to because Mum's just reminded them that they are a 'fussy eater'. However, whether your 'fussy eater' is six months or 16 years, in this chapter we'll guide you through some successful strategies that we have used.

REVIEW: TYPICAL FEEDING DEVELOPMENT TIMELINE

Let's start by remembering the typical timeline for feeding. We should be aiming to start solids no later than six months of age. However, if your little one starts solids at, say, eight months, then it is not realistic to expect them to jump straight into lumpy foods. This is like asking them to walk when they've not had any practice crawling or just balancing to stand up. Children need to move through the different developmental experiences to help strengthen and coordinate their muscles for different types of foods. Parents may purchase jar food to get an idea of the texture and consistency of first solids. However, not all jar foods are uniform in their consistency. Your child's feeding development has a large bearing on the food you choose from the grocery aisle. Choose according to your child's ability rather than the age recommendation on the jar. The jar assumes your child is going through the typical feeding timeline. With all things in life, few of us stick to the 'typical' timeline!

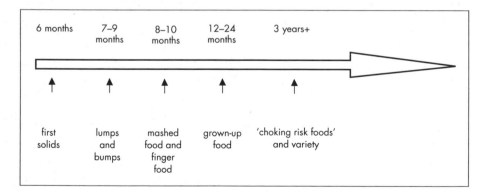

'HOUSTON, WE HAVE A PROBLEM . . .'—RULING OUT SOME COMMON SUSPECTS

Before we start, it is important to rule out some of the very common reasons why children may be fussy about food. First of all, let's establish that you have a problem. Ask yourself the following questions. Does your child:

- Seem happy most of the time?
- Generally sleep well?
- Have energy?
- Seem to be gaining weight and sticking roughly to their expected growth curves found in your *Child and maternal health baby book*?
- Seem to be active and interested in what is going on around them?
- Babble and make noises with their mouth (6–12-month-olds) or communicate using words (older child)?

If you've answered 'yes' to these questions, then allow yourself to relax! Feel free to read on and see whether some of the tips mentioned below can help improve food variety.

If you've answered 'no' for many of these questions, here are a few more things to think about. Start by ensuring that your child does not have any medical, structural or physiological reasons for food refusal or fussiness. Constipation is one such example. Dealing with constipation may improve your child's appetite. Chapter 5 discusses medical reasons for food refusal. It makes sense to treat the cause of your problem and not the symptoms; please have these seen to first.

The dinner meal is the most notorious for being diabolical for the 'fussy eater'. Ensure that you are providing your child with regular meals. We have lost count of the number of people who are convinced that if you starve a child at afternoon tea time, they will guzzle a huge dinner. In fact, the child is likely to take *less* at dinnertime. This hunger cycle information is discussed in more detail in Chapter 7. Also, check how close to the child's bedtime you are providing their evening meal. When we go to bed at 10 p.m., we are hardly likely to eat a huge dinner at 9.30 p.m., yet many parents seem to expect their children to eat at 6 p.m. before being bundled off to bed at 7 p.m.

Parents should also look at a daily food log and ensure that their child is not filling up on milk. By the time your child is 18 months of age, milk should be restricted to 500 ml per day (that's two cups). Yes, milk is good for them, but not as their sole source of intake. Excess milk intake contributes to constipation (see Chapter 5). We have included a profile at the end of the book so that you can more objectively look at what your child has each day. Filling this out once on a weekend and twice during the week can give you a good idea of your child's usual patterns. In cases where the milk-a-holic has emerged, the pattern can be seen very easily.

Let's return to our timeline now and visit our little ones at each of the major developmental feeding milestones for some new ideas on dealing with food fussiness.

SIX TO TWELVE MONTHS

At six months of age, many little ones are just starting their journey into food and eating. Although it should be a time of joy and anticipation, it is possibly every parent's worst nightmare. From the word go your beautiful baby fed well from the breast or the bottle; however, when offered solid food they went on a hunger strike (or, as many parents tell us, the 'air-only diet') and simply refused to have anything to do with food. What makes matters worse is that every baby you come in contact with appears to have their mouth permanently open and happily consuming the equivalent of a lamb roast meal at eight months of age. Feeding can definitely be a challenge; however, due to differences in children's needs, personalities, and rates of growth and development, there needs to be a simple guide to help the process and make it less stressful for all involved. Whilst the usual pattern of feeding development is discussed in detail in Chapter 2, we understand that many little ones have not read the instruction book and are playing well outside their parents' comfort zone! The following is intended to give you more information on what to expect and how to manage it.

Almost all babies starting solids for the first time appear to not enjoy the experience. They shudder, screw their faces up, possibly spit their food out or even try to swallow the mouthful whole. This often looks like a choking episode where Mum or Dad yank the little one out of the highchair and turn them on their end to remove what they think is an offending article. This can be a very traumatic experience for all involved, leading parents (and their baby) to believe the baby is not ready to start solids. The gagging is a completely normal reaction as babies have not yet learnt how to manage textures that are different to milk. The gag reflex is actually built in to our swallowing process to stop us from choking. Generally, babies between four and six months of age are losing or have lost their tongue protrusion reflex. This is where the tongue juts out of the mouth to help pull the nipple or bottle teat into their mouth. Now their tongue is ready to move the food around the mouth.

Allow children plenty of opportunities to have their hands in their mouth or to use their mouth to explore safe mouthing toys. These toys, like teethers, have lumps, bumps and different shapes. They provide a way for children to experience different textures in their mouth without the expectation of swallowing food. In babies the gag reflex is triggered from the front half of the mouth. With exposure to mouthing toys and placing their fingers in their mouth, they are able to desensitise this reflex and move it more to the back of the mouth. This is a necessary developmental step to allow them to move food around in their mouth without setting off the gag reflex.

The 'breastfeed-a-holic' or 'bottle-feed-a-holic' baby

For some parents, the fun begins simply with getting started on solids. Exclusive breastfeeding or formula will provide all the necessary nutritional requirements for baby until the age of 4–6 months. However, an over-reliance on breast milk or formula and a delayed or inconsistent introduction to solids is a common 'fussiness' issue for this age group. Fussiness rarely develops if solids are introduced and consistently presented at six months of age. Feeding from breast or bottle is certainly easier than learning the new skill of managing solids. As mothers we are biologically programmed to nurture, feed and protect our babies. It goes against our grain to withhold something we know is good for the child and that they are clearly signalling that they want (breast or bottle!). While breastfeeding remains an important part of their feeding regime, it must be supplemented with other food. It is for our children's own development, though, that we have to teach them to accept other forms of food and drink.

Well-meaning parents may try, on and off, to introduce solids, but, fearful of not providing their child with sufficient 'food' for the day, compensate with increasing numbers of breastfeeds or bottle-feeds, at a time when these feeds should be stable and gradually decreasing. At this age, children require more than just breastfeeds or bottle-feeds, and especially require a good source of iron, which is usually in the form of an iron-fortified cereal. Iron in the infant's diet is now important because the iron stores gained in utero have been depleted by about six months of age. Some babies consume a whole bowl of rice cereal whilst others are happy to have 1–2 teaspoons at any one sitting.

Do not add the rice cereal to the bottle as this will only confuse your little one. In addition, the rice cereal will make the milk thick and very difficult, if not impossible, to suck through a teat. Baby will become frustrated and may reject the bottle outright! Also, mixing rice cereal with milk in a bottle does not help them to learn to take food from a spoon.

If you find yourself in the situation where you have an 8- or 9-month-old who is exclusively breastfeeding and rejecting all solids, there is the 'hard-but-effective' technique. This technique is reserved for healthy babies. By this we mean babies who are a good weight for their age, who sleep well, who have happy and active periods during the day, who babble, coo and roll, and who have a good poo pattern (no constipation or diarrhoea) and frequent wees. Where the little one is a breastfeed-a-holic, it often works most effectively if Mum vacates the house for the day. Babies can smell breast milk and the looks and howls can be very hard for breastfeeding mums to bear. By all means express your milk to maintain supply, but enlist the aid of Dad, a partner, grandparent or good friend to feed the baby solids and expressed milk while you go through this one- or two-day boot camp. Remember a child will not willingly starve themselves and you will not have family services knocking on the door just by sticking to your guns! However, if food avoidance goes on for more than 24 hours, you may have to seek further professional help.

If your child is exclusively breastfed, ensure that you start the day with their usual breastfeed. Two to three hours later, their hunger cycle should have kicked in and they should be hungry. Use this hunger cycle to teach them that their hunger can be satisfied by food. Baby yoghurts or iron-fortified rice cereal mixed with a little apple or pear juice is a good place to start. Breastfed babies receive subtle variations and changes in their breast milk depend-ent on their mother's diet. Breast milk on the whole is somewhat sweet. As a learning exercise and to get things started, it is easier to offer a subtly sweet product to imprint the idea of food coming from a spoon as well as from the breast. Provide the usual number of feeds but no more if your child refuses solids. Once the child is taking 1–2 tablespoons of solids without fuss, it is the time to branch over to other flavours. The hardest part is getting the first few spoonfuls in. The information provided in Chapter 2 on early feeding and introducing solids is applicable once you have mastered the first few spoonfuls.

For children who are exclusively bottle-fed, there is less of a need for Mum to leave the house. This child is likely used to being given their bottle by a few carers and may not associate feeding purely with Mum. Use a similar approach to that described above for breastfeeding. Commence and end the day with the usual bottle-feeds. Use hunger cycles to help them learn the important association of eating and feeling full and content, and that this feeling can come from food as well as from a bottle. In both instances, it is very easy and very convenient for the child to take their nutrition via breast or bottle. They don't have to work very hard. Learning to take food from a spoon is work. But it is necessary work if they are to grow well and remain healthy.

Infant cues that they are ready for solids

Signs that baby is ready for more solid food include an interest in what other family members are eating or baby being unsatisfied after one or more milk feeds. It is not recommended to start solids before four months of age as babies simply don't need anything more than breast milk or formula and their little digestive tracts (guts) are still so immature. Babies between four and six months of age are not usually fussy; however, they can be *inconsistent* in their feeding whilst they are learning and developing the skills necessary to move the food around their mouth. This is often confused with fussiness. Trying very small mouthfuls (often as little as ¼–½ teaspoon) so they get used to the texture and feel of the food is essential, and it is important to remember that babies take time to learn to manipulate food in their mouth and also to learn to chew. The skills learned during feeding help to strengthen the tongue and allow it to explore the mouth. These are important developmental milestones which help with speech development as they get older. Being able to change your tongue shape is critical to making different speech sounds. If you give up and go back to exclusive breastfeeding or bottle-feeding beyond 6–8 months of age, children may be slow to develop speech and may also develop fussy eating habits by limiting the range of food textures they will try.

You will find little ones who seem to consume anything that is not tied down are usually more active, often boys, and are children who are generally more interested in food. Do not despair if you have a more reserved feeder, as this certainly does not mean that the little 'picky' eaters will not be getting enough. Your baby's weight, bowel habits and wet nappies will indicate if your baby is consuming enough food and liquids.

Six to eight months of age is a very important experimental time for babies. They are still consuming the bulk of their kilojoules from the breast or formula; however, this is an important time to offer new tastes and more importantly *textures*. We call this texture the 'lumps and bumps'. Many children that develop very fussy palates have often had their food vitamised or blended for far too long and reject anything 'lumpy'. If they turn their nose up at a lumpier vegetable or a more solid piece of banana, it won't be forever; they are just trying to tell you that they prefer the very soft, easier-to-chew-and-swallow version. It is up to you to keep offering the lumpier ones to develop their chewing techniques. Remember, a healthy, hungry baby will not starve itself. Having said this, some little ones do not seem to click into autopilot and learn to chew. Some of them need a little tutorial work. So we've included the following details, missing from many children's instruction manuals.

Spitting out lumps and bumps, or gagging on lumps

Children typically learn early chewing skills at about seven months of age. Often we will see children of about ten months or even 13–14 months of age who are spitting out lumps. This is because they have not got the hang of chewing. Children who pass whole pieces of food in their nappies have not chewed them (think corn and sultanas). There are a couple of ways of teaching your child to chew. These methods are often used simultaneously. Learning to chew is a relatively quick process once you have the know-how.

As we saw in Chapter 2, the tongue needs first of all to know what to do with the lump. One way of teaching this skill is by using a toothbrush trainer. Toothbrush trainers or 'first toothbrushes' can be found in pharmacies and the baby aisle of many grocery and large general stores. Toothbrush trainers have a handle at one end and a rubber tip at the other end. Some toothbrush trainers will have little lumps on the rubber and some of them more closely resemble soft thick rubber bristles. For our purposes, start with one that has lumps on the end. Place the toothbrush trainer into you child's mouth and guide it over to their gums, closest to their cheeks. Biting happens with the teeth at the front of the mouth, but chewing happens with the teeth along the sides and towards the back of the mouth. By putting the toothbrush trainer onto the lower gum, natural reflexes take over and the jaw will start to move up and down in a chewing action. The tongue, being very curious, will come over to the lumps and bumps on the toothbrush trainer to see what they are. This is where the magic is. The tongue's curiosity at wanting to investigate those lumps gives it practice at coming over to the gums. It finds the lumps or bumps on the toothbrush trainer near the gums. With this practice, you are helping to teach the tongue that lumps and bumps belong over with the gums (and eventually the teeth). Secondly, while the child is practising the chewing action, there are no loose bits being broken off that they have to be concerned about. They get to practise the chewing action without the pressure to actually chew and swallow something. It is important to give both sides a turn to develop chewing actions. You can watch to see that your child's tongue is indeed searching out the toothbrush trainer. Remember to smile and provide praise when they do. You can also 'show them' what to do by moving your jaw up and down in a chewing action too. This little exercise can be done once or twice a day and should take no more than 1–2 minutes. Do not, however, give your child a toothbrush trainer while driving in the car! Within a week you should notice an improvement in chewing abilities.

After a couple of days of using your 'chewing stick'/toothbrush trainer, you can start adjusting the texture of your child's food. For apple puree you can crumble in some Milk Arrowroot biscuit or shortbread biscuit. The crumbs need to be very small. The mouth is very sensitive and will seek out big lumps and remove them (or 'spit them out') as a safety precaution if they don't know what else to do with them. On day one you could start with your usual amount of smooth puree and a separate bowl with a tablespoon of smooth puree mixed with half to one teaspoon of the biscuit crumbs. Offer two spoonfuls of smooth, then one of the grainy mix. Remember to mime the chewing action and smile as your child copies you. Now that they've practised with their toothbrush trainer, you may also start to see them moving the grainy mixture to their gum ridges at mealtimes. Go back to the smooth and offer another two or three smooth spoonfuls, and then another grainy one. If tolerated well, try one smooth spoonful followed by one grainy spoonful and so on. The goal is to transition over to the grainy texture, and then to increase the size of the crumbs.

It is important to remember that this is a learning phase. We are giving the child the skills they need to start chewing. We are aware that there is limited nutritional value in the biscuits. The aim here is to provide the physical skills to manage food textures. This is done by using particular food textures. We are able to change to a full nutritional focus once the child has all of their chewing skills in place.

The following table provides some ideas on different types of purees and suitable 'grainy or lumpy' additives.

Table 8: **Food textures for introducing lumps and bumps**

Step 1	
Adding texture to savoury purees	Grated cheese; <u>fine</u> breadcrumbs; well cooked risoni or pastina (small pasta—available in the pasta aisle or baby food aisle); mashed pieces of avocado
Adding texture to sweet purees	Crumbled pieces of shortbread biscuit; mashed pieces of tinned fruit (pear, mango); mashed pieces of fresh fruit (banana, mango)
Step 2	
Increasing texture added to mashed savoury purees	Rice; pasta; shredded ham; shredded chicken; well-cooked mince with large pieces broken down with a fork
Increasing texture added to mashed sweet purees	Grated apple; mashed pieces of tinned fruit (peach, pear); mashed pieces of fresh fruit (soft pear, rockmelon, pawpaw)

The muscles needed for chewing are present, but will need practice to become strong enough to manage all the different types of food textures that we need to eat to keep us healthy. Raw foods like apple and carrot take a lot of chewing power. It's like trying to lift a 10 kg weight when you've never lifted anything more than a block of butter (250 g). We use foods of different textures to increase the strength of the muscles and their ability to manage hard, crunchy and chewy foods. Table 4 (on

p. 35) contains the progression of food textures from soft through to hard and crunchy. If we stick with the gym analogy, you need to work through the easy weights before progressing to the larger and heavier ones. This principle holds true for the jaw muscles.

Stuck on 'jar food'

Some parents or carers may choose to use commercially available infant foods. This can be due to a number of reasons such as being time-poor for cooking and pureeing, or for convenience factors. Home-cooked foods offer your child the best nutrients and truest tastes and textures and should be used whenever possible. If time is the enemy or they just didn't graduate as 'Suzie Homemaker', some parents will reach for commercially available jar food. Some mums can be very distressed that the hours they have spent cooking and blending are unceremoniously spat out while their cherub happily takes jar food. You will hear over and over again that babies have very bland palates. Certainly they have many more tastebuds than we do and so what may appear mild to us may set off fireworks for them, but take everything, including advice, in moderation. If you seem to have a sensitive little soul who prefers the bland flavour of jar food, gradually introduce them to your cooking. Carefully ensure that the texture of your food is not radically different from that of the jar food. Sometimes it is a texture issue, rather than a taste issue, that is causing the problem. Use a gradual approach by adding one teaspoon of your food into seven teaspoons of the jar food and gradually swing over the ratios. Once you've reached a 50:50 ratio, you could provide a few tastes with the 'Mum + jar' blend and then a spoonful of Mum's puree. Again swing it so that by the end of approximately four days you have converted your child to your own cooking.

What about increasing food variety?

Just as we have seen that we need to be persistent with introducing lumps and bumps, we also need the same stamina to keep dishing up other foods such as yoghurt, custards, cheese, meats, chicken and fish. Giving little ones their own small spoon or very soft fork can help them with their hand-to-eye coordination and many enjoy (or demand!) the responsibility of helping to feed themselves. Babies do not need teeth to chew soft lumpy food. Many breastfeeding mums have been on the receiving end of their little one's strong gums; however, having a few teeth will help with harder-to-chew foods such as tougher meat, chicken or dissolvable crackers. Children will need to be proficient with soft foods and soft chewable foods before moving onto harder, crunchier or chewier food textures. Foods can quickly become a choking risk if the child does not have the chewing skills for that food texture. Chapter 1 guides you through the different types of food textures.

By eight months of age, babies should have been exposed to other foods including lentils, baked beans, hommus, soft meats, chicken, fish, egg, cheese, custard and yoghurt. If meat is not a favourite by itself, try it as mince mixed into a pasta sauce or made into rissoles. Often meat, chicken and fish are rejected as they are tougher to chew, can be dry on their own, or break into multiple bits in the child's mouth. These are experiences that many children do not enjoy. Adding meat, chicken or fish to a sauce or using minced meat or chicken can make it more palatable and the mouth-feel more tolerable. Meats such as lamb shanks, or salt-reduced corned beef that has been boiled for a few hours, become quite soft and are often more popular as 'first meats'. It is important to include an abundance of variety for taste, texture, colour and smell at this early stage to ensure that babies and toddlers remain inquisitive and eager to try new things. Within each food group there are a number of alternatives that can be used if your child is being stubborn. For example, hommus (made from chickpeas) or baked beans are a great alternative for meat as they are high in protein and iron. More ideas on alternative foods to try when foods are rejected can be found in Chapter 3.

Between eight and 12 months, babies should be offered finger foods. Pieces of fruit and soft vegetables, muffins, pikelets, small sandwich squares or toast are ideal. By now water or milk from a cup should be a familiar routine. Many of the 'introduction to solids' books talk about keeping fruits, vegies and meats separate. This is a good place to start to watch for reactions indicative of food reaction or allergy. However, once you've established the relative risks, it is advisable to introduce your child to your usual meals, modifying the texture of the meal to match their oral development skills. So if spaghetti is on the menu, reserve a quarter of a cup, puree or mash it, and have it ready for Junior's lunch or dinner the following day. This reduces the amount of work in having to prepare multiple meals and also introduces your child to the family menu. Many handheld blenders make this process so much easier than the large food-processor varieties.

By 12 months of age your baby should be enjoying the family's food chopped or mashed. Of course, there are some foods that could prove a choking risk, such as whole, raw or undercooked pieces of carrot or apple, whole peas and popcorn, and these should be avoided for obvious reasons (see Table 3 on p. 30).

'It's not you, it's me . . .'—Parents' mindset and expectations

The key is not to become fixated on trying to completely balance your child's diet too soon. Provide as much variety and ensure that babies are progressed onto firmer foods regularly to ensure that there is a smooth transition to adult consistency by about 12 months of age. Using the tips outlined above, many children will be able to transition more easily through their lumps and bumps, then fingers foods and on to grown-up foods. However, if there appears to be a major problem with the mechanics of chewing in these early stages, then it is best to see a qualified professional for further investigation. A full developmental review with your child's paediatrician is a good place to start. Your paediatrician will be aware of feeding milestones. Due to their understanding and expertise with the speech mechanism, some speech pathologists also have specialist experience with infant feeding. Speech pathologists that specialise in infant feeding are often located in major children's hospitals.

Often, though, simple strategies can go a long way to improving the situation.

Children learn from us all the time. So, as with talking, waving and walking, they learn to feed, eat, chew and drink from watching you. In Chapter 1 we navigated the introduction to solids. Strategies such as smiling when your child accepts a taste to their mouth sounds simple but is important. Children like people smiling at them and often reward you by returning a smile back. This simple 'reward' helps to reinforce when they are doing what you'd like them to do. Frowning, saying 'no' or turning away are behaviours your child will not like. These strategies can be used when food is tipped off the highchair, for example, to discourage behaviours.

Avoid bringing toys to the highchair. Parents seek to distract their child by giving them a toy to play with, hoping that their child will just keep opening their mouth like an automated doll. When the interest in the toy wanes, the parents frantically search for the next toy that will hold the child's interest for the next 4–6 spoonfuls, and the endless loop cycle continues. There are a couple of good reasons for not even venturing down this path.

First of all, mealtimes are about eating and social exchange. When adults sit down at a dinner table and one of them brings a newspaper, that person takes themself out of any conversation and social exchange. They are absorbed in their own affairs. Bringing a toy to the table distracts the child from eating and stunts the development of the social exchange that happens at mealtimes. Talk to your child about what they are eating, what it looks like, what it feels like, what it smells like.

Secondly, by distracting the child, they are less in tune with what their body is telling them about chewing and about feeling full. At this early stage the mouth is learning to chew like a new chopping machine and the special feedback loops shoot up to the brain for checking to make sure the machine is doing a good job. The brain can send 'quality control' messages back to say that the food has not been chewed well enough to safely swallow it down, and to keep chewing. The brain also has connections with the stomach. The stomach has stretch receptors to let us know when we are full. It is important for children to learn to listen to their body to know what this sensation feels like. As parents, we need to learn to trust our children and their signs that they are full. Some of these themes have been investigated in regards to childhood obesity.

Provide small tastes often. If you can get a smidge of sweet potato up to your child's lips or just into their mouth, smile and provide praise. If the child spits it out, make no comment—certainly no gasps of horror or admonishing of naughty behaviour. These behaviours from you are more likely to evoke more spitting from the child. Think of new flavours as a bit like getting into a cold pool. You might go up to the edge and put your hand in and then move back. Next time you might put your toe in and then pull back. Then put your toes in and move them around a bit. After that you might step into the water for just a moment and then clamber out. Finally, you might stand on the step and paddle about. Who knows, after that you might just leap in! Taking new foods is very similar. Each step of the process can be fun, thrilling or anxiety-provoking for children. Taking it a step at a time helps them to feel safe and confident. They need a calm and patient coach to help them learn their way. So if you get a taste of sweet potato onto their lips and they lick it—it's a win! Place a smidge into the side of their mouth. The child may take one or two small amounts to start with—this is a win! Regroup and try again the next day. Calm, confident persistence is the key. A German proverb states that patience is a bitter plant but it bears sweet fruit. If you try to leap too many steps ahead, your child will soon let you know that they are out of their comfort zone.

If attempts at solids have been such a disastrous affair that the mere sight of a highchair is enough to send your little one into full flight, it might be time to try a different setting. Try taking a picnic rug outside, or sit on the floor, or sit on a verandah or deck. Have your own bowl and try to entice your child to have some from your bowl rather than trying to feed them from their bowl. Some children do not like having things 'done to them', for example, brushing their teeth. One way around this is to let them be part of the feeding process by feeding you. You can show them mouth opening and sounds of happy eating and then feed them. For the very independent child you can help them to feed themselves by using hand-over-hand feeding. They hold the spoon, you place your hand over theirs to collect the food and guide it into their mouth.

ONE TO THREE YEARS—TRYING NEW FOODS AND CONSOLIDATING OLD FOODS

By about one year of age the goal is to be cooking one meal for the family. Your child's meals are likely to need modification to ensure that the textures are appropriate for their chewing skills and the sizes of the pieces are appropriate for their little mouths. We remember one mum giving her 12-month-old a piece of broccoli the size of his fist and complained that he wouldn't eat it. Breaking it into small florets that would easily fit into his mouth, he happily wolfed the lot. If you can transition at this point to 'one meal for the family' you are likely to save yourself loads of time, effort and energy in the years to come.

Twelve to 24 months is possibly the toughest time of a baby's food calendar. The mighty toddler by now has made up his mind as to what he will and won't eat. This age is still too young to negotiate with them as they don't have the cognitive processes required for this. Some fussy eaters you will recognise by their appetite (or lack of it!), some seem to be colour or texture specific in their food preferences, and then there are the defiant ones who simply say 'No!' Let's start with appetite.

Toddlers usually fit into one of the three categories below:

- Category 1: 'Happy with the same thing for every meal for the rest of my life.' These tykes are not happy with change; however, appear to have a balanced, if somewhat boring diet.
- Category 2: 'Will eat anything you give me, happy to try new things and very satisfied after each meal.' You will also find this little one rummaging around in other people's lunch bags or taking food out of the hands of other children. Usually an 'always balanced' diet.
- Category 3: Gradually reducing their intake to 'safe foods' such as plain pasta, rice crackers, milk and Vegemite sandwiches. Will not try anything new and may get so anxious about the introduction of a new food that they can sometimes spontaneously vomit. This diet is always going to be unbalanced.

The first two categories can provide a perfectly balanced healthy diet for a growing toddler; however, Category 2 is more ideal as they are happy to move with the family's tastes and willing to try many new things. The more variety, the less chance of nutritional deficiencies.

We tell parents to aim for a benchmark of 15 different food types or varieties for their child to consume within a 24 hour period. Table 9 below is an example.

Table 9: **Varieties of food within a 24 hour period**

Meal	Food	Varieties of food offered at this meal
Breakfast	Weetbix, milk, pear	3
Morning tea	Crackers, cheese, avocado	3
Lunch	Bread, margarine, cheese, Vegemite	3
Afternoon tea	Yoghurt, banana, sultanas	3
Dinner	Pasta, tomato-based sauce, grated carrot, corn, mince	5
Snack	Apple, yoghurt	1
TOTAL		18 different foods—Sounded hard, but usually do–able!

Toddlers that fall into Category 1 concern parents and health professionals long-term as they run the risk of becoming bored. This leads to rejection of foods, followed by an unwillingness to replace foods with an appropriate alternative. For example, you have the little guy who loves peanut butter sandwiches. However, after a year of the same sandwich he decides he doesn't like it anymore, or, worse still, his kindergarten tells you not to pack anything containing nuts, and he doesn't want anything else in its place. Over the year he has not been encouraged to try other fillings and becomes upset and anxious about the unknown. Over time his intake can soon resemble Category 3 so it is important to expose young children with their developing tastebuds to a plethora of tastes and textures. Remember, don't be limited by your own likes and dislikes; your child could be the next king of brussel sprouts!

If you happen to have a toddler who launches into their second year of life with only a handful of foods they like and trust, then you do have your work cut out for you. The first line of defence is making the diet as balanced as possible to provide the necessary nutrients for growth and development. (See Chapter 3, 'What is a good diet?'). If their diet is poor, then a vitamin or mineral supplement may be necessary whilst you encourage them to expand their food repertoire. If sickness, mechanical/chewing difficulties, anxieties or any other medical reasons have been ruled out, then it may come down to shear stubbornness on your toddler's part. See 'The defiant non-conformist' (p. 105) for more information on these little warriors.

Introducing a new food

If you are having trouble working out the shortfalls in your toddler's diet, seek help from an accredited practising dietitian (APD) in your local area who can provide balanced menu plans specifically designed for your child. However, if you are generally happy with your child's growth but they seem to be refusing one or two particular food groups, the most common being fruit and vegetables, then it is about trying to introduce these foods in a fun interesting way.

Kate recalls, 'Back when my daughter was about 16 months I enlisted the help of my 4½-year-old son who happened to be a great eater at the time. She had decided that pasta was the order of the day, week and month and was not going to have a bar of any-thing else put in front of her. Prior to this she would happily try something new. We had been playing tenpin bowling on the kitchen bench whilst I was preparing dinner. The pins were still set up when their plates were put in front of them. My son happily cruised through his meal whilst my daughter refused to even take a bite. They were still excited from the game of bowling so I used this as a non-food incentive. If she took a bite she could have a go at bowling. My son happily ate and bowled until it drove my daughter to distraction. She couldn't bear not having a go and finally relented, taking a bite. The meal (a zucchini slice) has since become one of her favourite meals. The key is getting them to at least try it in such a way that you are not using other foods or sweet rewards (such as ice-cream) to do so. It is also important not to use language such as "If you don't eat this you won't watch TV". It is a much better tactic to take the attention off them and reward them when they make the right choice. Often children play to negative attention and conform when this is removed.'

Whilst trying a new food seems like a very sensible idea to most parents, children rarely take the same point of view. We also have to remember that while we are 'experts at eating and trying new foods', our children are novices. Would it surprise you to know that there are at least seven steps to trying a new food? For adults, these are so ingrained and automatic we don't even think about them. At a fruit shop we pick up our peaches and feel them for firmness (touch), we bring them up to our nose to take in their aroma (smell). Now all of this happens before we've even paid for them and start eating them! Following is our 'automatic guide' to trying a new food. Some children just need to be shown the road signs.

Steps for trying new food

Choose your food depending on your child's comfort zone. For Category 3 children (the 'white food child'—see p. 104), it may be best to start with a food that is very similar to one that they currently take. For children with the basics, increasing their repertoire can be done with the aid of food textures and bridges shown later in this chapter. For a practical example, let's start with something like apple. For some kids the first step can be just touching the food!

Julie usually starts with two plates and a whole apple. She asks the child what the apple looks like. She asks them to touch the apple (skin on, in its whole form). Walk their finger over and touch it. We are aiming to make this fun. She then asks them if they have big strong muscles in their arms and to show her their arm muscles. She picks up the apple and lifts it with both hands over her head. Then she asks them to show her that their muscles are strong enough to do that too. Then she lifts the apple with one hand and swaps over to the other hand to show that each arm is strong. Again she asks them to do the same. At this point she takes a knife and cuts the apple in half. They talk about what the inside of the apple looks like and the outside. She touches the inside and then it is the child's turn to do the same. They talk about how the outside of the apple is dry, but the inside is a bit wet. Then she lifts the apple and smells it and puts it straight back down again. She does the same thing again and then asks the child to do the same. Use lots of smiles and positive encouragement. Let the child know that they have touched and smelled the apple and that you're finished. Put the apple away and give cuddles or read a story or have a play afterwards to reinforce that this food stuff is a positive thing. All sessions need to be short (five minutes). We also recommend doing it at a time *other than* mealtimes.

On day two you can briefly revisit the touching and smelling of the apple. Again have two plates at the ready. Take the skin off the apple while the child watches. Cut the apple into quarters. Now cut three slivers of apple from one of the apple quarters. Place one sliver on each plate and put the rest away. Notice how big the plate looks and how small the apple sliver looks. Julie usually tells the child she's going to do something funny. She picks up the apple sliver and gives it a kiss. She does it again and then asks the child to have their turn. Aim for three kisses. Use your fingers to show the child each turn. Stick to your rules. If you say three, that means three, not four, five or six. This is where you build trust with your child.

The lips are very sensitive to texture. By bringing the food to the lips they can feel it, experience the sensation briefly and have it end. Repetition allows for desensitisation and getting used to the food. For children who are very defensive, you can start further away from their mouth. Start with touches to the cheek or the chin, and once successful then move to the lips.

The tongue tip is also very sensitive to both texture and taste. Now we pick up the apple sliver and lick it. Use the same idea as above by taking turns. Then we 'do magic!' Pick the apple sliver up, hold it between your teeth (but don't take a bite) and move your hands away whilst holding the sliver between your teeth with a 'tah–dah' (hands out) type action. Take the sliver back out of your mouth and put it on the plate so that the child can see that you have just held it with your teeth and that is all. Now it is their turn. If things are going well, you may wish to progress. If it has been a cautious exercise, it's time to stop for the day. Put the apple away, let them know that they have done a great job and are finished, and give lots of smiles and hugs or read a story, give tickles or play a game.

Repeat the process from the previous day so that you have your three little apple slivers. Remind them of 'doing magic' or ask them to do one of the steps that is very easy for them to give them some confidence. With the third sliver of apple, cut it so that you have little pieces that are about the size of your little fingernail. Let the child know you are going to hide one of these pieces in your cheek. They need to close their eyes while you put it in your mouth and then guess which side it is on. Open your mouth to show them where it is. At this point Julie makes a big deal that her teeth have found that apple and want to chew it, so she chews it, and then swallows it down. You can repeat this process, 'hiding' the apple on the tooth surface of the other cheek. Then it is their turn. If they manage to get it in but do not initially chew, that's okay to start with. Encourage them to use their big teeth to squash it down. The pieces are deliberately small so that the sensation is not huge. By placing the food on the teeth, you avoid relying on the tongue to place it on the teeth. There are pressure receptors on the teeth that encourage chewing, but the teeth are far less sensitive than the tongue or lips as far as food texture is concerned. This makes it an ideal 'hiding place' for a new food. Aim to repeat this part three times so that they have eaten three little pieces of apple. Again keep it fun. Phrases like 'Where did you put that apple? Is it in your pocket? Where did it go? You didn't chew that did you? You didn't swallow that did you? How amazing, where did it go? Do you think we can do it again? I wonder if we can do it at the same time? Let's show Daddy/ Grandma this special trick.' If they have succeeded let them know that they have eaten some apple. Their body will thank them because it loves that apple to help it grow. This also lets them know that they are doing it for themselves—not for you. Give them lots of praise and hugs and finish your game.

Now that they have had the opportunity to place the small morsel of food directly into their mouth by avoiding their pressure-sensitive areas of the lips and tongue, it is now time to re-engage these areas. On your next session, you can progress to using the whole sliver and encouraging them by still taking turns to take a 'mouse nibble' and then a 'shark bite'. You may wish to read Chapter 1 on taking a bite, as for many toddlers this can be a 'work in progress'.

Having successfully held, kissed, licked, chewed and bitten the new food, you are ready to introduce the food into meals or snacks. It must be kept achievable, however. So, to start with, place a piece of apple sliver on the child's morning tea plate along with two other things you know they will eat. This is also where behaviours and rules become established. Julie's children know that she expects them to take a bite of foods on their plate. If they choose to have more, that is fine. If they choose not to, then there is nothing else to eat until the next meal or snack. So if at this point you remind your child that this apple sliver is just like the one you've had all that fun with, they should be happy to at least take a mouse nibble or shark bite. Remind them though that they've also eaten a sliver before, that it is easy-peasy, and that their body thanks them for it.

If your child is very wary, you can take a different tack. Kate's example of her son and daughter and their tenpin bowling game illustrates this technique beautifully. Find a game your child enjoys. Age-appropriate toys and games are listed in the table below. Bring the food out and put it to one side and engage the child in the game. It must be a game where you need to take turns though. Once the child is firmly entrenched in the game, start the processes as above, with the child needing to complete a lick in order to have their turn. Keep it short, sharp and fast. Make sure you are involved as well. Provide the model, and take your turn of the game. Now it's the child's turn. They get a turn for each step of trying the new food (touching, kissing, licking, etc.). Again these sessions should only last for about five minutes. End with the usual praise and reward for things that the child has done.

Table 10: **Toys and games to aid in learning to eat new foods**

Child's age	Possible toys or games
6 to 12 months	Smiling! When they try a lick, a taste, a tiny smidge, a bite.

Child's age	Possible toys or games
12 months to 3 years	Blowing bubbles; placing puzzle pieces into a shape sorter; getting the next puzzle piece for their puzzle; getting the next piece of track to build the train track; pushing the button on a toy that makes a noise or pops up.
4 to 6 years +	Plastic bowling game, taking turns at board games (e.g. Snakes and Ladders, Trouble, Guess Who?). Make a visit to a speciality gift or toy store to see which games or activities peak your child's interest and use these.
Other tips	Borrow a toy from a friend for a week to keep the toy or game 'special'. Join a toy library to keep variety fresh without the expense of purchasing new toys.

Patience and perseverance are the next two ingredients. Once the apple sliver goes down well, gradually increase the size of the 'sliver' so that over the course of a few days it becomes a quarter of an apple. When it is time to move from one quarter of an apple, provide the one quarter and a sliver. Gradually alter that sliver so that you have two quarters, and so on. When the change is gradual, it doesn't seem like it is changing much at all.

Realistic expectations are so important from us as parents. Julie recalls, 'It took my 5-year-old son the better part of two months to progress to eating a quarter of an apple at school. To begin with pieces of apple would boomerang from home to school and back again untouched on a daily basis. We had worked through all the steps at home and he would eat some apple for morning or afternoon tea. Then it was time to transition from having it at home to having it at school. We went back to an apple sliver in the lunchbox to keep it achievable. In the early days I would ask him to open the container at school and see what was in there so he could tell me when I picked him up. He knew to bring home what was not eaten so that I could see what he had had for the day. One day I placed a few sultanas in the container with the apple and let him know there was a surprise in there to entice him to open the container. I asked him to tell me what the surprise was and to have a bite of the food. Hunger got the better of him and he ate the lot. We built up from that sliver to the apple quarter and so on.

'The first food was the hardest. Now we can run through the steps up to taking that fingernail-sized piece in one session. During the winter months he takes orange, mandarin, strawberries and sultanas to school. Using fruit that is "in season" means that their flavours are at their best. We have done the same with salad vegetables. To start with his plate would have a single baby spinach leaf, half a grape tomato and a slice of cucumber. He has discovered he likes salad dressing and also barbecue and tomato sauce. To start with he was allowed to dip his vegies in the sauces or dressing, providing a bridge to the new taste of the vegies. Nowadays he has a full salad on his plate, with no sauce, mayonnaise or dressing. He tells me he has made good choices for himself. He eats till his tummy tells him he is full and I am very conscious of not putting too much on his plate—if he's hungry he asks for more!'

Mouth stuffing—Making 'chipmunk cheeks' and then spitting the food out

Children may stuff their mouths for a couple of reasons. The food might taste so good that they just can't get enough. For example, children may stuff their mouth with lollies and chips. This is a choking risk and children need to be supervised and shown how to slow down and chew the food before putting more food in their mouth. At parties, this behaviour can appear when the child feels they may miss out if they don't keep up with other children. Providing children with a small bowl to put 'their share' of the goodies into is one strategy that can be used.

Some children stuff their mouths when their chewing skills are insufficiently developed. Some children require help to learn that you need a little bit of room in your mouth to manipulate and move the food around so that it can be chewed properly. These little ones end up with too much in their mouth and then, finding they can't manage it, spit the sticky mess out. Like most of us, they are unlikely to want to put the sticky mess back in and have another go. As parents, we dislike seeing the sticky mess and may chastise the child for being 'rude' or 'having poor manners'. What these children really need are some specific skills. Other mouth-stuffers leave food in their mouth for a while because they have worked out that their saliva softens it. Bread that becomes moist gets a bit smaller in size and with minimal chewing can be gulped down. This process is not, however, ideal. Gulping down great chunks of food places an unnecessary stress on the oesophagus, the 'pipe' between the throat and the stomach.

A quick reminder about bread—bread is not soft, it is fibrous. You cannot mash bread with a fork. When you pull it apart with your fingers, it doesn't disintegrate and easily fall apart, you need to use pressure. Some adults break their teeth on sandwiches. Bread requires as many chewing strokes as raw apple and even meat.[1] Children may initially seem to cope with bread, but if you watch closely they may be sucking on it, or holding it for longer periods in their mouth so that it becomes moist. Bread absorbs three to five times more saliva than pasta. Some children will also hold the sandwich between their teeth but then use the strength in their hands to tear the bread, leaving a chunk in their mouth. These children have not developed sufficient bite strength to be able to use their jaw muscles to help their teeth cut through the bread. Children need to learn to bite and *chew* bread.

For older children who have managed by moistening their food and largely swallowing it whole, there are some strategies to bring their chewing up to speed. Firstly, you can try the toothbrush trainer exercises mentioned previously in 'Spitting out lumps and bumps' (p. 82). Secondly, you can take little fingernail-size pieces of dissolvable foods and place them directly onto the gum/tooth surfaces. You will need to physically place them on the gum surface closest to the cheek. If you put the piece into the front of the child's mouth, you are relying on them to move the piece to the chewing surfaces. This is the skill we are trying to teach them.

What is a 'dissolvable food' and why use them when teaching an older child to chew? Dissolvable foods are dry and can initially seem hard. Think of an ice-cream wafer or a small piece of dry breakfast cereal. Some other dissolvable solids are: scotch finger, shortbread and wafer style biscuits, Cruskits, potato chips and Cheezels. When you put the ice-cream wafer or dry cereal in your mouth, it will 'crunch' when you bite it. This gives good feedback—you chew it and it makes a noise! But its texture changes quickly when you add moisture to it. Add saliva and it becomes wet and soggy. Not very many chewing strokes are needed to make this food soft and safe to swallow. It is agreed that its nutritional value is minimal, but its value in being an 'easy chewing food' is priceless.

To recap, by breaking the piece to a 'bite size' the child learns that there should be space in their mouth while they are chewing. By placing the piece onto the chewing surfaces, you are helping the child to learn that this is where food that needs chewing goes. By using a dissolvable food, you provide the child with something that will give them some feedback when they bite on it (the crunch), and needs few chewing strokes to break it down for safe swallowing. Bit by bit we can change the texture to increase the strength of the jaw muscles so that your child can manage a wider variety of foods and food textures.

Mouth raking

Some children will use their fingers to rake food or liquid out of their mouth. Some of these children are also the spontaneous vomiters. Keep pieces very small till you've overcome this stage. Once the food is in the mouth, clasp both of their hands (it's hard to rake food out when someone has your hands!) and swing them up to say hooray, or start a simple hand clapping game with them. The amount should initially be so small that it is barely detectable. Once achieved, move in small incremental steps back up to a normal portion size.

The timid observer or 'sensitive' child

This child is one who parents will readily identify. They may have been sensitive since they were little, fussing if they were too hot or too cold. They may be bothered by clothing tags, may dislike the feeling of grass or sand underfoot, may not like having their teeth or hair brushed, or may dislike having messy hands. For these children, these types of sensations seem to keep triggering the 'this is new' reaction. Over time and with repeated exposure most of us will get used to the sensation and it no longer causes a big reaction. For these little ones it either takes that bit longer for them to get used to the sensation, or their reactions are so strong that their parents protect them from the experience by avoiding it, therefore delaying their ability to get used to it. Julie recalls one mum whose little one was noise sensitive. This family had resorted to watching television with headphones or with no sound at all, in order for the child to sleep at night. Whilst this example relates to sound, the same sort of thing can happen with food. If the child's reaction is particularly strong, it may scare the parents. The parents are less inclined to try the experience again, and so the child does not have the opportunity to learn to adjust. Some of these children become 'white food children' (see the following section).

With timid children, the processes for trying new foods that have been described above are still appropriate. It may just take a longer amount of time and more patience. They may need to touch the food a vast number of times, or kiss it oodles of times, before they are ready to move to the next step. Perseverance is again the key. Avoid 'saving' these children by providing them with foods you know they will eat. Whilst they might eat marshmallow, chocolate wafers and chocolate pudding, it is not okay to offer these when your child refuses dinner to appease your guilt that they will go to bed hungry.

The 'white food child'

These are Kate's Category 3 children. As noted above, these children are the biggest concern nutritionally, because of their unbalanced diet. A 'white food diet' usually consists of milk, yoghurt, white bread or toast, chicken nuggets, chips and ice-cream. When Kate looks at this diet she sees a poor balance. When Julie looks at this diet she sees 'easy chew' food textures and predictable textures and tastes. The 'white food child' needs to be taught how to try new foods in addition to working on the stamina and strength of their chewing muscles. This lack of skills contributes to their poor nutritional balance because it limits the food textures they can manage.

Children who are down the 'soft and easy-chew' end need some practice with progressively harder, chewier or crunchier textures. But it can't all happen at once. Just as your child didn't become a fussy eater overnight, so too the process of increasing food textures and varieties will take some time. Think six to nine months of calm, patient persistence. Keeping a food diary can help when you despair that nothing much has changed. You will be amazed at how many new foods your child can try in a month if you keep your expectations in order. Julie recalls one session with a 'white food child', where the child had managed to go from touching to eating an entire sliver of pear in ten minutes. Mum's response was the 'reward' of more pear in the car on the way home and a whole pear in the lunchbox the next day. The expectation was too high. This child had just climbed to base camp and Mum was asking him to sprint up Mt Everest on the way home and repeat it the next day. His trust in the process was destroyed.

The 'defiant non-conformist'

They say variety is the spice of life and that if we were all the same it would be a boring world. However, there are some children born with an inbuilt ability to find our internal buttons and transform the mildest parent into a demented being. These children often need to have firm rules and clear boundaries. They will thrive on the 'traffic light system', where green always means go and red always means stop. If red sometimes means green, they will pull out every trick in the book to have things just the way they like them. Behaviour is a big part of the solution here. Let's look at this a different way. When we were growing up in the early 70s, a hat was a 'good idea' but often for appearances. In the days of skin cancer enlightenment, hats are a health must. Day care, kindies and schools have adopted the 'no hat—no play' philosophy. Children learn this rule quickly. They may not like wearing the hat, but they like to play more. It's the same idea with bath times and bedtimes; stick to rules and we all know what is expected of us and there are no disagreements. We don't let children stay up or go unbathed just because they have a tantrum, the same principle is true for food.

The key is to maintain a united front between all those who are involved in the feeding of your young toddler. There is nothing worse than having your set of rules undermined by Grandma or Uncle Tom who give in to your toddler's demands. They learn very quickly to stick to their guns when demanding something different for dinner. We believe that from 12 months of age children should be consuming the family meal (modified for texture, size, spice, salt or richness in taste if required), with the motto *'One family—One meal'*. Sometimes this requires us to dig our heals in slightly deeper than our beloved children's. Stick to your guns and offer up the family meal in a happy, quiet and engaging environment.

Eating with your children can help the process as they learn from and often copy you. If the meal is refused and a tantrum begins, remove the plate without fuss. Tell them they may return to the table when they calm down. If the meal is continuously refused then remove it; however, do not offer an alternative except for a small glass of milk before bed. Again, many parents offer up something different, believing that their child will starve if they go without. This is not true. A few skipped meals will not harm your toddler; however, learning to have a tantrum until they get the potato gems or fish fingers for the third night in a row will. Remember, there are very few adults who only eat potato gems and fish fingers for dinner!

In the Cichero household the children know that they are expected to take one bite of whatever is on their plate—the choice is then theirs: they can keep eating, or call it quits, knowing that there is nothing more on offer till the next meal. For children in the clinic, Julie asks them to take their turn in the 'learning new foods' activities, but if she strikes resistance, she asks once more. After counting to three in her head, she calmly says 'You haven't done what I asked—please stand over there', pointing to a spot about two metres away, but where she can still see them. She waits for about 30–60 seconds (depending on the age of the child), and then in a happy chirpy way says 'Thank you, would you like to come back now?' Then it is straight back into the fun of the game or taking of turns—there is no talk or admonishing for naughty behaviour. The most she has ever had to repeat this process in a single sitting is three times. Again, patience and persistence is the key.

At the dinner table, congratulate them if they take their bite. After that, let them sit for the remainder of the meal while everyone else finishes. Talk about what happened during the day or something that you are looking forward to. Remember that meals are supposed to be a social exchange. If you don't talk about the food or what's still on the plate, it loses its 'status' as the dynamite that makes Mum cry or explode.

The 'spontaneous gagger or vomiter'

Some children have honed the art of saying 'no' to a diabolical point where they will spontaneously gag or vomit. These are tricky times. Some of these children may not have the vocabulary they need to communicate with you that they are feeling distressed. As babies or toddlers, at some point these children may have closed their mouth or turned their head away and gave lots of non-verbal cues that they did not want what was on offer. If their loving parent did not recognise these cues and continued on regardless, the vomit is one sure-fire way of getting your attention. So rather than use their words, some of these children go straight for the big guns. For other children, the inside of their mouth is super-sensitive. Some of these children may not have had the opportunity to have their hands in their mouth or to put toys into their mouth while they were babies, leaving the gag reflex far more easily activated.

It is important for all children to learn to communicate, so providing them with words to describe not only foods but how they are feeling is important. Often these children are frightened. Once they are frightened, vomiting comes very easily to some children. Now we may not see the situation as one that invites fear, but for a child without the toolkit to try a new food and take it in very small manageable steps, it can be a scary experience. However, if you've identified that they are feeling frightened, then the next step is to make them feel more comfortable, rather than abandoning the process. Taking them gently through the steps is a must. You may even have to move through the steps with a food they are familiar with so that they understand each part of the process.

With all gaggers and vomiters we provide a firm 'No—that's not okay'. We also let them know there is no vomiting in this room. To begin with only, you can also encourage these children to breathe through their mouth to reduce the intensity of the aroma of the food. But, once the child has been able to manage three times in this fashion, it is time to remind them to breathe normally so that they continue the process of getting used to all aspects of the food (texture, taste and aroma).

THREE TO SIX YEARS—BATTLE OF THE MINDS

This age group, despite what some parents think, is a much easier age to deal with. They at least have some understanding of food and its use, and usually some good communication skills. The older children, especially around six years, will often start eating something because someone has told them that it will make them run fast or make their hair shiny. The key here is finding what makes your child tick. If you have a girl who loves brushing her hair or having you paint her nails, use this as a way of teaching her about the foods she eats, especially if she doesn't drink a lot of milk or consume other calcium-rich dairy foods. Explain that the yoghurt in the fridge contains special things to give her strong nails or that the chicken in the stirfry will help make her hair longer and shinier. This concept worked well with a 5-year-old boy who refused to eat fruit. Kate told him that all fruit contained little things called fighter pilots to help with his immune system—which would help fight colds. If he didn't get a cold he could play his weekend soccer, his one true obsession. Well, his father rang Kate that afternoon reporting that his son had consumed four pieces of fruit in the two hours following their appointment. Again, it is finding something that children are passionate about.

For the children who are of the defiant non-conformist variety mentioned earlier, harder line tactics may be required. For these children, the antics are much more fun than having a healthy body. Many times these children will respond to working towards a special event. For example, some children at the clinic loved going fishing, others loved going to the park, for others it was books, etc. The rules were set: We're going to try some new foods this week (using the behavioural approach), and effort on the child's part resulted in activities that they enjoy. We encourage parents to find a reward where the parent and the child participate together to strengthen parent–child bonding. This approach can backfire in a big way if the goals are beyond reach or the parents' expectations are a burden. For example, the 'white food child' who was offered a puppy if he completely changed his diet in a fortnight, and the child who had a piece of that watermelon for Julie so then it was immediately a permanent feature of his lunchbox.

It is very important to talk to your children to find out exactly what it is about a certain food that they don't like. Many children talk about slimy textures or too hard to chew or too floury or bitter. Occasionally a child will reject a whole food group after one bad experience. For example, an overripe bruised banana in the lunchbox can taste bad and give off a strong smell and can cause a child to completely go off fruit. It is important to take them to the fruit shop and show them what else is on offer and get them to select something they would like to try. Providing a variety of options and explaining that the banana was just bad luck is essential for maintaining their trust and confidence in you. It is also worth mentioning that children between three and six years will start to develop likes and dislikes. We all have favourite foods and the ones that we dislike, so it is worth acknowledging this when discussing food choices with your child. Often, we come across a frustrated mum whose children will not touch their greens only to find out that 'Dad thinks they are disgusting too'. Maybe Dad can work through the new foods program with their child. United we stand!

One particular stand-out was a child whose diet consisted of chocolate, chocolate biscuits and milk. This child was quick to temper, hyperactive, had limited communication, and on the verge of being referred for medical tests for autism or attention deficit hyperactivity disorder (ADHD). It emerged that the child worshipped his father and that his father had the same diet. Brave Mum made them go cold turkey. The house was emptied of the chocolate and chocolate biscuits, cola, etc. and these were replaced with healthy foods. There were howls of protest when the child pulled open cupboard doors and the refrigerator and realised what had happened, but Mum stuck with it and he very quickly learned to eat healthy foods. Lo and behold his behaviour, attention and communication also improved to the point where medical assessment for a disorder was no longer being considered. Sound too good to be true? Try living on your child's diet for a week and see how you feel . . .

MORE THAN SIX YEARS—FEARS AND PSYCHOLOGICAL ISSUES

At this age a fussy child (avoiding whole groups of foods or not willing to even lick a piece of watermelon) is usually harbouring a great deal of fear towards food. This can be as a result of many different factors including sickness such as severe tonsillitis, delayed solids as a baby, severe constipation or a bad experience with food. It can also be as a result of inconsistent rules from parents or caregivers. Often out of complete exhaustion many parents give in to demands when their children are young only to realise that it has been happening for years, laying down the foundation of a fussy eater. A 6-year-old needs firm guidelines once all medical reasons for food refusal have been eliminated. You need to gently explain the dining rules of the house—not unlike bedtime and teeth-cleaning rules, which are usually non-negotiable with parents—and stick with them. The backlash from this age group is usually more severe, although improvements to the diet appear to happen more quickly as the consequences (no dinner) are understood. Remember, a child will not deliberately starve themselves. Reward your child for even the smallest change as it shows their willingness to at least try. The main thing at this age is not to revert back to old habits if it appears to be an uphill battle—kids have stamina. Having realistic expectations is also critical. You need to be prepared for at least six months of being consistent with the way you deal with refusal, and consistent in providing the food you want your child to eat, to see the changes happen. Your child did not wake up fussy one day, it happened over time, and it will take time to reverse the situation.

It is in your own interest to work through this difficult period because one child's behaviour can suddenly have a domino effect on brothers and sisters. One family that Julie treated had Tom (an 11-year-old) who was a fussy eater and Fred (an 8-year-old) who had been a very good eater until he realised that Mum would cook different meals for the older child. Suddenly, Mum's problems multiplied as the 'good eater' started employing the same strategies as his older brother. The boys used extreme gagging to reduce Mum to tears. Who would want to repeat that process every night? Mealtimes had definitely become a battle. This family responded very well to the steps for introducing new foods. A few steps were modified, such as touching the food up to the lips rather than kissing it, after the first few times. Licking the food became just touching their tongues to the food in a discreet way. Tom surprised himself on a number of occasions as he turned to his mum and said, 'Actually I kind of like this one'. She was also far more responsive to him when they came across the few foods where he said, 'I really can't stand the way that feels in my mouth or the taste of this food'.

Tom and Fred also became more involved in menu planning for the week. Each child was asked to choose a meal for the week. The rules were always the same: You take a bite, if you choose to have more that's fine, if not, that's fine too, but there's nothing else. Mum stood her ground when the inevitable whingeing started, kept her cool and dished up meals. The boys had lost their reaction and the family was well on their way to their biggest goal of eating out at a restaurant together as a family.

HELP! MY CHILD DOESN'T EAT . . . ANYMORE

Kids change their minds all the time. They may eat VitaBrits for 364 days of the year and on the very last day will announce that they hate VitaBrits which throws parents into a state as they also tell you they don't like anything else either. The same story has been played out with sandwiches in school lunchboxes, breakfast with bowls of porridge left untouched and wheat biscuits soaked in milk. Chapter 3, 'What is a good diet?' has some great tips on what to do when children are avoiding entire food groups. Apart from this, it is time to think outside the square. Below we tackle some of the more common 'but he/she won't eat . . .' topics we've seen.

'Won't eat anything but white bread'

This tip came from a bakery. If you are trying to convert your child to wholemeal bread, try making the sandwich with their favourite filling using one piece of white bread and one piece of wholemeal bread. The effect is a checkerboard. The combination of the two breads allows the child a gradual transition. Ensure that fillings are favourites at this stage to avoid rejection on two fronts. It is quite easy to transition over to wholemeal sandwiches after this. The same principles can be used with moving from wholemeal to grainy bread.

'Won't eat sandwiches anymore'

There are lots of different ways of providing 'breads'. Try bread rolls for example. Dinner rolls can be just the right size for children to eat, and still have time to kick the football around at school. Tortilla wraps and mountain breads can also provide a fresh change. Use the opportunity to take children to the grocery store or bakery and check out the different types of breads and rolls that are on offer. They are more likely to eat something that they have had a choice in. 'No' to sandwiches might just be 'Please Mum, sandwiches are okay for three days, but I need something different for the other days'. A tin of baked beans put into a child-friendly container or the occasional boiled egg can change things a bit. Freeze little homemade pizzas or the occasional homemade sausage roll with all those great vegies in them to be included as a lunchbox surprise. More tips on lunchboxes in Chapter 9.

'Won't eat porridge/wheat biscuits anymore'

Children are allowed to get bored and request change. Try providing a new cereal without milk for them to try in a tiny serving bowl—like a taster. Children often transition to new cereals by eating them dry first. This is not a problem. Just let them have their glass of milk beside it. There are no rules to say that you 'failed breakfast' because you didn't drown your cereal in your milk. If cereal is just not your child's thing, you may have a little continental eater. Try boiled egg, some grated cheese and strips of ham or chopped chicken. Offer some toast, some fresh fruit, yoghurt, French toast or even an omelette if you have the time. Think outside the box.

FOOD TEXTURES AND BRIDGES

Whilst parents often think that taste is the culprit for food rejection, in many cases it can be the texture that the child finds challenging. Some children prefer certain food textures to others. For example, your child might prefer 'dry foods' while 'wet/moist' foods are rejected. Children who prefer dry foods can be 'bridged over' to wetter textures by using dipping sauces where wet and dry are used together. You can start by asking your child to dip the end of their finger into the sauce or dip to taste it (after they have first smelled it). They can work their way up to dipping dry food into wet food. For some children with heightened oral sensations, the feeling of wet and slippery yoghurt or the unpredictable movement and texture of scrambled eggs can be enough to cause them to gag. Some children, over time and with repeated small exposures, may eventually become accustomed to wet and unpredictable food textures.

We commonly refer to foods by name and give little thought to their many other qualities. We use many senses when we eat food:

- Vision: What does it look like? (shape, colour)
- Olfaction: What aroma or fragrance does it have?
- Touch (hands, fingers, lips, tongue, teeth): What texture does the food have?
- Taste: Does it taste sweet/savoury/bitter?
- Hearing: How does it 'sound'? Is it crisp and crunchy?
- Mouth sensation: Does it feel creamy/warm/cool/irritating?

Foods can be described in terms of their chemical and physical properties. Chemical properties include the food's taste, smell, whether it dissolves in water, and its colour. Physical properties include size, shape, stickiness, roughness, toughness, whether it is composed of particles, and how easy it is to change its shape (deform it). Here are some adjectives to describe foods: Hard, soft, brittle, chewy, gummy, powdery, flakey, woolly, lumpy, fibrous, light and fluffy (aerated), crisp, rubbery, spongey, smooth, rough/course, pasty, creamy, watery, soggy, sticky, tacky, greasy, stringy, melt–in–your–mouth, slimy, mushy, sharp/harsh (astringent).

In the following table you will find some suggestions for transitioning children over to new foods. As bridges, they are *temporary* measures that should be phased out over time. These are teaching tools to make the transition process to the new food as smooth as possible.

Table 11: **Food bridges**

Goal	Suggestions
Introduce more vegetables	Use familiar flavours to tone down the new flavour.
	Use sauces (tomato, barbecue, mustard, taco sauce), dips (hommus, tzatziki), light sour cream, mayonnaise.
	Begin by keeping vegetables separated on the plate.
	Begin with raw salad vegetables—peel and de-seed cucumber, choose the less acidic grape tomatoes, choose spinach leaves for iron, include orange pieces, use a peeler to peel strips of carrot.
	Steam vegetables such as broccoli, carrot and asparagus, then proceed to corn, beans and peas.
Introduce more red meat	Begin with soft, mild-flavoured meats such as chicken, beef mince in a mild sauce or fish in a light sauce. Encourage children to chew bread crusts to develop the chewing muscles needed for meats.
	Introduce simple, mild-flavoured casseroles with few or no vegetable chunks and small meat pieces.
	Step up to tender cuts of beef or lamb, or pork cutlets (lightly score pork cutlets with a knife to make it easier to break up).
	Cut pan-fried, baked, grilled or barbecued meats into small pieces (once your child is 6–7 years of age they should be able to cut their own meat with some direction and practice).
	Use sauces and marinades to improve the flavours.

Goal	Suggestions
Introduce more fruit	Children who like 'dry' foods and don't like wet or sticky hands: • Begin with grapes, sultanas and fine slivers of apple. • Move on to mandarin as it is dry on the outside. • Dry banana by rolling it in fine coconut and serving on toothpicks. • Wet fruits can be eaten with a fork or toothpick. Children who prefer 'soft' foods and already enjoy fruits such as banana, watermelon and strawberries: • Encourage them to chew bread crusts to develop the chewing muscles needed for more fibrous fruits. • Cut hard and fibrous fruits into thin or small pieces. Children who prefer 'savoury' foods: • Try fruits with simple flavours such as apple, orange, mandarin, dried apricots, sultanas and pear. Cut fruit into pieces rather than serving as whole fruits.
Introduce different-looking food (e.g. sushi)	Begin with sandwich wheels using a familiar filling to introduce children to a different way of presenting foods and a different way of holding and eating foods.
Introduce fish	Try crumbed fish for the child who prefers dry textures. Add mild sauces to enhance the flavour. Serve salmon and tuna in patties or mornays.
Introduce egg	If your child doesn't like eggs: Begin with French toast as a bridge from a familiar food. Step up to an omelette—cheesy flavourings can disguise the egg flavour and the texture is not as off-putting as scrambled eggs.

Goal	Suggestions
Introduce dairy	Milk—children who are unsure about milk from a cup can be introduced to it using mildly flavoured milkshakes or fruit smoothies. Then step them up to a glass of plain milk.
	Ricotta and cream cheese can be cooked into savoury and sweet dishes to provide dairy in less obvious ways.
	Yoghurt, custard and cheese—if they don't like the mouth-feel of yoghurt or custard, they will probably still get dairy from cheese or milk.

EXTREMELY RARE CASES OF 'FUSSY EATERS' FOR SPECIAL CONSIDERATION

Over the years we have seen some very different reasons for food refusal. Some children have had a very traumatic food experience in their toddler years; like the child who was physically force-fed an avocado sandwich by a childcare staffer. This child displayed behaviours at home that showed the depth of his emotional scarring from this episode, such as hiding behind cereal boxes whilst eating food. His visit to the clinic was prompted by an upcoming school camp where a teacher had caught wind of his restricted diet and was keen to 'help' this child overcome his fears. Fear emanated from this child at the mere mention of the camp. This one episode had ramifications some eight years after the initial event and will probably follow him for the rest of his life. Never, ever, force a child to eat food. The consequences are diabolical.

A teenager had been studying the human digestive system. She had been made aware that we hold our breath to swallow and there is a common passage for food and breathing. She had somehow convinced herself that she was going to 'get it wrong' and would end up with food going down the wrong way. Hence, food that needed chewing became the most anxiety-provoking for her. Her 'new' diet consisted of yoghurt and chocolate. Her change in dietary textures and variety, however, had also produced weight loss because she was no longer getting the right amount or types of food. The teen years are a very difficult time to negotiate in terms of body image. This episode certainly was a difficult one for her to rationalise. Prior to seeking help with her eating, her parents had already organised to see a psychiatrist, as there were other behaviours that had become a concern. This was fortuitous. Her issues with the way she was thinking about chewing and swallowing and the self-talk in her head were best managed by the psychiatrist. Julie was able to show her how her swallowing system worked and demonstrated using water swallows that her body would automatically protect her airway. She was able to show the teenager that her mouth and throat muscles were in good condition and behaving as they should. With this knowledge, she was able to work with her psychiatrist to change her self-talk.

In another rare case, the child in question had a choking episode on a piece of meat. The experience caused a fright, but the situation was highly charged because it happened on a parent access weekend. Mum was upset about what happened and berated Dad for being careless. The 6-year-old quickly determined that food was dynamite and could be used to gain extra attention. She altered food textures and food variety almost immediately, which resulted in rapid physical effects such as weight loss, fatigue, lethargy and difficulty concentrating. For the grown-ups involved, the food also became the subject of heated debates. Having determined that the girl had no physical problems with swallowing, the family was referred to psychology services for counselling.

Fortunately, cases such as these are rare. They bear mentioning, however, as a reminder of how small things can escalate.

Medical reasons for food refusal

We've established that it can be quite normal for children to be 'fussy' around food from time to time. An old family friend used to say as we'd moan about the latest thing our children were doing to test our sanity: 'Don't worry it's JAP'—'just a phase'. There comes a time though, when even the most laidback parent will become concerned. At these times, it is important to seek medical advice to ensure that there is not an underlying medical reason for your child's food fussiness or food refusal.

This chapter covers some of the most common medical reasons for fussiness around food. Many parents battle with the delights of constipation and reflux. Teething, tonsils, food allergies and intolerances are also common culprits for medical or physiological reasons for food refusal, rather than the child's sheer bloodymindedness! Knowing and understanding how our body's hunger cycle works and how this affects their food fussiness can be like a revelation of biblical proportions (it was for Julie!). Pleasantly enough, it is one of the easier issues to manage! There is also a small but significant group of children who start life with extra challenges that also contribute to feeding difficulties. Premature infants, children with cerebral palsy, and also those with heart and breathing problems may all have some difficulties with feeding.

In all cases of food fussiness and particularly food refusal, it is important to rule out any medical or physiological reasons for their behaviour. Treating the medical or physiological cause of the problem will see far greater returns than battling on against the issue, which experience shows is unlikely to correct itself without help.

TEETHING

Let's start with the most contentious 'reason' for food fussiness! Even before the excitement of first solids, the eruption of the first tooth is a much-anticipated event the likes of which it seems entire folklore has been written about for nearly 5000 years.[1] In 18th-century France, half of all infant deaths were attributed to teething. Thankfully, medical science has put that particular association to bed. Teething can variously be distressing or an absolute breeze for parents and their offspring alike. The first tooth generally arrives at about six months of age but can occur as early as birth or as late as the child's first birthday.[2] The full complement of 20 teeth is generally present by 30 months.[3] So, on average, you can look forward to one tooth erupting per month between six months and 30 months of age! In a study of Australian parents it was concluded that teething was distressing not just for the infant but also for the parents. If you are at all concerned about delays in teeth coming through, consult your local dentist. The generally accepted signs and symptoms of teething are shown in the following table.

Table 12: **Signs and symptoms associated with teething** (adapted from McIntyre & McIntyre, 2002,[1] and Wake, Hesketh & Allen, 1999[3])

Signs	Swollen gums where the tooth is erupting (intra-oral ulcers)
	Facial flushing (red cheeks)/rash around the mouth
	Drooling/dribbling
	Gum rubbing/biting/sucking
	Ear pulling or rubbing on the same side as the erupting tooth
	Nasal congestion
Symptoms	General irritability—crying and crankiness
	Disturbed sleep patterns (wakeful)
	Change to bowel patterns (especially loose motions/diarrhoea)
	Loss of appetite
	Increase in body temperature (up by about 0.5°C compared with normal temperature in the three days prior to tooth eruption)
	Sooking

Some parents, child health nurses and GPs may diagnose 'teething' when there are few other explanations for the child's change in routine or behaviour. Generally, babies are most irritable when teeth are breaking through the gums, and back teeth seem to give children more grief than their front teeth. Equally, you will come across medical, nursing and allied health professionals and even other parents who will tell you that 'teething pain' is a load of poppycock.

From a medical perspective, the child's immune system is being pushed into gear between about six and 12 months of age, due to the loss of maternal immunity that was bequeathed to the child via the placenta in utero, and then during breastfeeding. The argument here is that the child is dealing with small blips of very mild infections that are firing up its immune system and displaying the symptoms we have come to associate with teething. It is possible that the small breaks in the gums where the teeth are coming through allow bacteria and organisms a site of entry to the child's developing immune system that was not previously available. While this explanation makes sense, Julie can clearly remember the eruption of her 12-year molars: 'I had felt quite unwell with temperatures, loss of appetite and awful headaches for a few days. I clearly remember the feeling of the broken skin in my mouth and feeling the teeth emerging amongst the gums. My children, on the other hand, have all had their six-year molars arrive with nary a complaint!'

Symptoms of teething may appear and disappear over several days. Giving a very wide margin for individual variation, teething has been reported to have an eight-day cycle. Irritability may be present for the four days before the day of emergence of the tooth or the three days after the tooth has erupted.[1] However, having all the symptoms of teething will also not necessarily guarantee you of the production of a tooth!

There is also something to be said for our very individual levels of pain tolerance. One man's wince is another's mighty howl. However, an overdependence on teething as the get-out-of-jail-free all-encompassing response to all behaviours is not helpful. The teething symptoms reported above have been noted by good quality sources and published in respected journals. If symptoms are very severe or persistent, it is imperative to consult your GP to rule out other medical conditions. High temperatures (38.8°C and higher) in particular must not be ignored or put down to teething. High temperatures could indicate that your child has an infection (e.g.

ear infection) or other serious illness that deserves prompt medical attention. Wake and colleagues[3] in their interview of 92 Australian parents found that a substantial minority of parents attributed potentially serious symptoms (e.g. high fever, smelly urine) incorrectly to teething.

Management for teething

Management of teething is associated with keeping pain under control, cooling the gums and providing lots of love, assurance and care. Teething gels provide a local anaesthetic (lignocaine-based products) or analgesic to help ease the pain. Ensure hands are washed and clean before applying teething gel to the baby's gums. Infant paracetamol preparations deal with pain at a whole body (systemic) level rather than local level and also address temperatures. Ensure that the appropriate number of doses per day is followed, as for both local and systemic medications too many doses can cause toxicity. McIntyre & McIntyre[1] reported a case of a child who was overdosed on a teething gel where the contents of three tubes had been applied in a 48-hour period! Note that ibuprofen (aspirin) is not recommended for the treatment of teething. We can be very thankful that treatments such as leeching the gums and lancing an 'x marks the spot' into the gum over the likely eruption point have melted into the pages of history.

Chilled teething rings can be used to soothe swollen gums. Pain relief occurs due to the pressure on the gums when chewing the teething ring. Gently rubbing the gum can also provide temporary comfort. Chewing on fingers and teethers also stimulates the production of saliva. It is advisable to wipe the excess saliva from your baby's face to avoid the development of a rash around the mouth and on the chin which will only contribute to further discomfort.

In regards to treatment for teething, there are some old wives' tales that need to be put to bed. Putting a baby to bed with a bottle will not improve their teething and is more likely to increase their chances of dental decay on the newly erupting teeth. This is due to the constancy of the milk bathing the teeth while the infant sleeps with the bottle in their mouth. Similarly, adding sugar, honey or jam to feeding bottles will increase the likelihood of dental decay and will not address teething issues. For these same reasons honey-coated pacifiers are also off the menu.

Finally, if it seems that your little one is teething, graciously accept that they will be off their food for a short time. They will let you know when they are ready for food and will likely eat with gusto to catch up.

CONSTIPATION

From mouth to anus is a very complex series of pipes and plumbing which all have to work in unison if digestion, absorption and excretion is going to work effectively. If one step is interrupted, then the whole process can come to an abrupt halt—literally. If a little system becomes constipated, for all sorts of reasons, this can have a direct effect on their appetite. It's kind of like a train track network. When one train leaves the station this allows the next to follow in line; however, if one train is delayed on the platform, then no other train can enter the station. This brings the whole transport system to an abrupt standstill. This is a similar scenario to constipation.

Your little one's bowels are happy when undigested fibre and dead bacteria combine together in the gut and make up a nice soft stool. This travels happily through the gastrointestinal system where it is finally excreted as a bowel movement, stool, poo, poop or number two. Each family has their own toilet language, especially around toilet training time when a bowel movement is the number-one topic of conversation for the day! If the stool is too small or too hard or pebbly, then it may not move efficiently, causing constipation. The poo then becomes drier and larger, effectively becoming stuck in the system. This has a *kick-back* effect as the stomach doesn't empty properly when nothing is moving below. If the stomach remains full, then there is no appetite, and the child often shows no desire to eat and is labelled 'fussy' or 'picky'. This may lead to more serious problems such as impaction or fear of going to the toilet. The keys are the right ingredients in the diet to start with and a relaxed environment.

What causes constipation?

Firstly, it is important to understand how the body digests the food, absorbing what it needs and then packaging the leftovers in such a way that the body can happily get rid of them. When we eat we start to digest some foods in the mouth. We have the enzymes present in our mouth to start breaking down some foods such as bread, cereal, rice or pasta. The food is chewed and mixed with saliva and then swallowed where it enters the stomach for digestive juices to be added to break down the food further. The stomach keeps the food here for as long as it is needed, before releasing it into the lower intestine where further breakdown and the absorption of nutrients happens. After the intestine absorbs what the body needs, the leftovers enter the large intestine where they are bulked together with other particles such as dead bacteria. Water is reabsorbed into the gut which causes the stool to become drier, firmer and darker as it travels along its final path before being excreted. *Constipation* is a term used when the body cannot excrete the leftover waste products effectively, causing straining, pain and often bleeding from the bowel. This can happen for a number of reasons, addressed as follows.

Breastfeeding and formula feeding

It is quite normal for babies to poop infrequently whilst they are being exclusively breastfed or bottle-fed. They can happily fill their nappy after each feed or as little as once every seven days. Their little guts are still very immature and can't cope with large particles of fibre until they are at least four months old. Breast milk and formula contains no fibre, therefore there is not a great deal left for the gut to process into a stool. A breastfeeding baby may only poo once every three to four days which is *not* constipation. However, if the poos become very pebbly or the child appears to be distressed when trying to move their bowels, they may need extra feeds or water to provide more fluid. See your GP, dietitian or child health nurse for advice on numbers and amounts of feeds and fluids.

Starting solids

The transition from breast milk or formula to solids can change a baby from a 'pooing' machine to a blocked drain. This can be due to the introduction of solid foods which adds bulk to the gut, or the addition of more iron to the diet. Both of these slow things to a crawl. Constipation at this age can be very distressing and painful to the infant who may suffer cramping, irritability and bloating and often have a decreased appetite. Try to increase water and mashed or blended fruits to provide natural softeners to help speed up the movement.

Not enough fibre

Constipation in older children is often a result of not enough daily fibre or water.

Fibre comes in two forms: soluble and insoluble fibre. Soluble fibre is the soft dissolvable fibre found on the inside or flesh of fruit and vegetables, some oats and wholemeal flours. This fibre is important for health and especially cholesterol-lowering; however, due to its dissolvable nature it does not add bulk to the stool. The insoluble fibre found in fruit skins, most vegetables, nuts, seeds and wholegrains is made of cellulose and is completely indigestible to the human intestinal system. Only some mammals such as sheep and cows with four stomachs are designed to break down this fibre.

It's the insoluble fibre that the body cannot digest and this, therefore, ends up as residue or roughage in the gut. This roughage gives bulk to our stools and helps us defecate. If your little one does not like the skin left on fruit, avoids vegetables like the plague or hates the 'bits' in their bread, then the chances are they may not be getting enough fibre to help things move through their system. The amount of fibre required by children is shown in Table 13 below.

Table 13: **Daily fibre requirements**

Age	Amount of fibre per day
1–3 years	14 g
4–8 years	18 g
9–13 years	20–24 g
Adults	30 g

Ten grams of fibre is not difficult to achieve. This can be done by encouraging a few pieces of fresh fruit, dried fruit, wholegrain or wholemeal breads and crackers, and a few serves of vegetables or salad items during the day. Table 14 gives some examples of typical amounts of fibre in everyday foods.

Table 14: **Typical fibre amounts found in everyday foods**

Food	Quantity of food	Fibre amount in this quantity
Apple	1 whole	3 g
Pear	1 whole	4 g
Dried apricots	4 halves	1.5 g
Wholegrain bread	1 slice	2 g
Wholegrain cracker	4 small	2 g
Vegetables	½ cup	3 g
Salad	½ cup	2 g
Breakfast cereal biscuits	2 biscuits	4 g

It is quite common for young children to have a poor fibre intake as many are not happy to chew through skins on their fruit or pick through the 'grainy' bits in their bread. A typical *low-fibre* diet looks like Table 15. Compare this with a *fibre-enriched* diet shown in Table 16.

Table 15: **Typical *low-fibre* diet**

Breakfast	Bowl of Rice Bubbles plus milk
Morning tea	Rice cracker with cheese
Lunch	Vegemite sandwich plus apple juice
Afternoon tea	Pikelets and jam
Dinner	Spaghetti bolognaise followed by yoghurt
Total fibre: 4 g	

Table 16: **Fibre-enriched diet**

Breakfast	Bowl of wheat cereal plus milk
Morning tea	Wholegrain rice crackers and hommus
Lunch	Wholemeal or high-fibre bread plus cheese and tomato
Afternoon tea	Fresh fruit
Dinner	Spaghetti bolognaise with grated carrot, peas and corn followed by yoghurt and chopped strawberries
Total fibre: 20 g	

It is important to encourage children to get used to wholegrains, or, as we have often heard them referred to, the 'little nutty bits' in their food. Wholegrains offer many health benefits, not only providing much-needed fibre but also antioxidants, omega-3 fats, and some vitamins and minerals. Getting children used to edible fruit and vegetable skins is important to help boost their fibre as well as vitamin intake. Many vitamins and minerals are found only a few millimetres under the skin and can often be removed when the fruit or vegetable is peeled. Try chopping the fruit into small bite-sized pieces or threading onto toothpicks or skewers to encourage children to consume the skin. Cutting grapes in half to expose the flesh can encourage chewing as the child can see and taste the inside of the fruit. Fruits such as mandarins and oranges have pith around each segment which is insoluble fibre. This is another great choice to bump up the fibre. Blending fruits into yoghurt or milk smoothies helps to pulverise the hard-to-chew bits whilst still maintaining their presence. Sometimes a bit of smoke and mirrors goes a long way! (See Chapter 6.) Dried fruit is another great way of increasing the fibre in your child's diet. Dried sultanas, currants, raisins, apricots or prunes can be eaten straight from the pack or baked into foods such as pancakes, pikelets, scones or bread.

Fibre supplements are readily available from chemists and supermarkets; however, it is important to check with your GP or dietitian regarding the use of these with young children. As a general rule fibre supplements are not recommended for children under the age of five years. For older children they can be handy for bulking up the diet. There are some powdered fibre supplements on the market that are colourless, odourless, tasteless and mix completely clear into water, which is very handy if you have a very stubborn 6-year-old who is not consuming enough fibre. The key is to still encourage two pieces of fresh fruit, five half-cup serves of vegetables or salads, plus wholegrain cereals, breads and crackers daily. If they are becoming constipated it is best to get the whole system working as it has a direct flow-on effect to their appetite.

Not enough water

Water is the main ingredient to help soften stools. Think of a sponge in the kitchen sink. When it dries out, it shrinks and becomes quite firm. As soon as you put it in water, it softens and expands. This is a bit like what happens to our stools in the gut. If we don't drink enough water or available fluid during the day, our poos become quite firm and dry like the kitchen sponge. Children are no different, and we have to make sure they are drinking enough throughout the day to keep their stools soft and moist. Babies and very young children need approximately 125 ml of fluid per kg of bodyweight per day. This roughly equates to 1250 ml for a 10 kg child. The older child requires 40–60 ml fluid per kg of bodyweight per day. Water is absorbed from foods such as fruit, vegetables, milk, custards, yoghurt and soup as well. Children should be offered only milk and water throughout the day, paying particular attention when living in warmer climates.

A note on the milk-a-holics (see Chapters 3 and 4): Often children who are addicted to cow's milk and consuming large quantities suffer from constipation, as well as iron–deficiency and lack of appetite. This is usually due to the fact that they are not having enough fibre and bulk in their diet because they have no appetite or desire for other foods. For children over the age of 18 months, reduce their milk intake to no more than 500 ml per day. This will give them an opportunity to feel hungry and consume greater variety in their diet.

On a non–dietary note, it is important to encourage good toileting habits from an early age as it is common for children to become constipated due to fear of going to the toilet, or lack of routine, or lack of time to sit on the toilet after a meal. It is not uncommon for children to 'feel the urge' during or immediately after a meal. At toilet-training time, parents feel like referees, coaches and motivational speakers all wrapped in one. It's important to congratulate your young son on his wonderful achievement as you both stand over the toilet bowl staring down at his contribution to the city's sewerage system! A healthy diet, adequate fluid and active lifestyle need to be coupled with a relaxed 'pooing' environment to encourage healthy bowel habits.

REFLUX

Difficulties associated with reflux will draw as many different opinions as those related to teething! The past ten years has seen a lot of information and treatment for infant reflux emerge. Reflux has been associated with difficult and fussy feeders. Reflux or regurgitation is a normal part of the growth and development of babies. In fact, almost 75 per cent of babies under four months of age suffer from reflux.

To fully appreciate what reflux is all about, a quick review of the anatomy of the feeding apparatus is necessary. Between the throat and the stomach there is a tube called the oesophagus. The oesophagus has a valve at both ends. When we swallow, the valves open to allow food/fluid to pass through the oesophagus and into the stomach. The valves close to keep the food/fluid in the stomach and prevent it from re-emerging into the throat where breathing is usually happening. In all infants under 12 months of age, the valve between the throat and the oesophagus is weaker than it is for adults. For efficient feeding the infant uses a lot of tongue power to draw the fluid from the breast or bottle into the mouth and push it into the oesophagus. If the valve between the throat and oesophagus was very strong, it would make the feeding process very difficult and likely result in back-flow. Consequently, this valve and the one between the oesophagus and the stomach are 'looser' to allow for efficient transport of the milk to the stomach. But on the flip side, these 'loose' valves can allow fluid from the stomach to flow back up into the oesophagus and for spitting-up after feeds. Reflux occurs when the sphincter between the oesophagus and the stomach allows stomach content to flow into the oesophagus. Reflux can happen when the valve is relaxed and there is reduced muscle tone. However, it can also happen when pressure in the abdomen (tummy region) is high (e.g. when the baby is crying long and loud!) and forces the valve open.[4]

Reflux happens in all infants to some extent because of this unique physiology. Unlike vomiting this response takes no effort and generally does not faze babies at all. We often refer to them as the 'happy chuckers'. Generally the symptoms of reflux resolve as baby gets older and the gut becomes stronger. Sometimes reflux completely disappears once baby is able to sit up by themselves, can stand up or starts on solid foods. Adding bulk to the stomach using more solid foods or using different infant formula can make for a more stable stomach and less likelihood of liquid being propelled across the room when baby burps.

There is no need to do anything if your baby is happy and developing well, although you may want to have a few dozen shirts and drop sheets on hand for yourself. Sometimes, however, reflux may be due to some underlying medical issue that may need to be investigated.

Severe reflux left untreated can lead to a very stressed mother and baby and feeding problems down the track. If you are concerned, the first stop is your child's GP or paediatrician who can advise you on the best treatment for your child.

Other reasons for reflux symptoms

As noted above, the way babies are anatomically set up predisposes them to reflux to a great extent. 'Reflux' babies also tend to be unsettled little ones. It is important to watch for your baby's cues to pick up when they are hungry before they are howling the house down. Crying in itself increases reflux episodes. In order to have a long loud cry your baby needs to take in a good lung full of air. In doing so, they use their diaphragm. This is a very strong muscle that separates the ribs and thorax from the tummy (abdomen) area. As they take in their lung full of air, their diaphragm pushes down on their abdominal cavity and increases the pressure there. Provide some feed and if they are very worked up and continue crying, the milk will pop back up very easily, making baby uncomfortable and fussy during the feed. Milk that flows too fast or too slow can also unsettle a little one and this may cause them to cry also. Problem-solving the cause of their distress is important. A lactation consultant or child health nurse can assist with the problem-solving. Learning how to settle your baby so that they sleep well is also important so that signs of tiredness are not misread for hunger signals. Some tired children will feed and fall asleep, while others will rebel, and if forced to feed will start to dread feed times.

Severe reflux

Some children present with reflux due to abnormalities of the oesophagus and also problems with stomach emptying. This group are thankfully very small in number. Some groups of children are more at risk of severe or 'pathologic' reflux. These include infants with prematurity, congenital heart disease, oesophageal disorders, tracheo-oesophageal fistula (hole allowing unnatural connection between the oesophagus and the trachea, leading to the lungs), brain tumours, neurological problems, cystic fibrosis and bronchopulmonary dysplasia.[4,5]

Reflux becomes a matter of concern when it causes breathing problems which affect the airway or lungs, or feeding problems resulting in failure to gain weight and thrive. However, breathing problems are also obviously related to difficulties with the breathing system. These need to be attended to in a different way than if the breathing difficulties were a result of reflux. Consultation with your GP or paediatrician is imperative for any breathing difficulties noted. It is the doctor's role to determine the cause and treatment of the breathing problems. This is not an area to muck around with.

Table 17 lists the breathing problems and feeding problems seen with severe reflux. Of these, the most significant for diagnosing true pathology, in order of significance, includes: frequent vomiting, failure to gain weight and grow, snoring/snorting (stertor); blue discolouration around the mouth (cyanotic spells), and choking or gagging.

Why do children become so distressed with severe reflux?

The stomach has acid to help to break down food particles. When stomach acid mixed with stomach contents flows back up into the oesophagus, it can cause pain or discomfort. The stomach has a special lining that allows it to tolerate the acid. The upper part of the oesophagus and the throat do not have this special lining and the acid can burn these structures, particularly if it happens numerous times per day. There are also special sensors (receptors) in the uppermost part of the oesophagus. A bit like a safety switch, if refluxed material reaches these sensors, an automatic ejection response is activated.[7] The vomiting reflex quickly accelerates the liquid away from the throat and the entrance to the airway.

Table 17: **Signs and symptoms associated with severe infant reflux** (adapted from Morgan & Reilly, 2006[6])

Breathing problems associated with reflux (not part of the normal infant experience)	**Feeding** problems associated with reflux (not part of the normal infant experience)
• Noisy inward breath (stridor) • Snoring/snorting (stertor) • Wheeze • Cough • Nasal congestion • Hoarse voice • Blue discolouration around the mouth during or after feeding (cyanosis) • Fluid enters the lungs (goes down the wrong way) • Breath holding associated with refluxed material entering the lungs (going down the wrong way) • Airway closure associated with refluxed material entering the lungs (going down the wrong way) • Pneumonia	• Frequent vomiting during and after feeds • Choking or gagging during or after feeds • Back arching • Drooling • Irritability during feeding • Wet burps • Difficulty gaining weight

Treatment for reflux

Any severe or ongoing difficulties with reflux should always be investigated and treated by your GP or paediatrician. Reflux can be treated in a number of ways. Parents are often advised to keep their infants upright after feeds for about 20 minutes. Gravity assists with draining the oesophagus. Note, though, that seating the child can make matters worse. Poor muscle tone in the trunk can increase pressure on the tummy and make reflux more likely to occur. Parents should strive for short, frequent feeds. Sucking on a pacifier or clean fingers after a feed has also been found to be helpful. Sucking helps to stimulate saliva which has natural antacids in it. The sucking also stimulates the oesophagus to empty.

Positioning sleeping infants so that the head of the cot is raised higher than the foot of the cot has also been suggested. But there is no real evidence to support this practice. Lying infants prone, on their tummies, has been found to be helpful in reducing reflux. This helps with tummy emptying, and reduces energy expenditure, crying time and likelihood of material entering the airway (aspiration).[4] Bear in mind that sleeping while lying prone is not recommended due to increased risk of sudden infant death syndrome (SIDS).

For some time the practice has also been to thicken milk feeds to make them more dense or heavier. This method relies on physics, being that a heavy liquid is more likely to stay in the stomach than a light liquid. However, the research literature does not fully agree with this practice and warns that the thickener can cause difficulties with absorption of calcium, iron and zinc, particularly if the thickener is mixed with infant formula.[5] Thickening of feeds probably grew in favour following parental reports that reflux symptoms dissipated when infants started first solids, most commonly rice cereal. There is possibly a happy coincidence that the introduction of rice cereal happened when the infant's oesophagus and other oral and throat structures had also grown, strengthened and matured. Rice cereal should not be introduced before four months of age as infants do not have the skills to safely swallow it. Rice cereal should not be added to milk in a bottle as it is too difficult for the infant to extract it through the teat.

Reflux can also be treated under the guidance of medical prac- titioners using drugs. Medications such as omeprazole (e.g. losec and others) have been used to prevent stomach acid production, while other medications simply neutralise stomach acid. Note, though, that reflux will still occur. However, the refluxed material will no longer be acidic and, therefore, less likely to cause pain and discomfort. For very severe cases, surgical options may be explored. The most common of these is the Nissen fundoplication, where a small portion of the upper part of the stomach is wrapped around the lower part of the oesophagus and stitched into place to create a stronger and tighter band at this point, helping to keep stomach contents in the stomach. Surgery is reserved for very serious cases where all other medical avenues have been unresponsive and the disease has been unremitting beyond 18–24 months of age.[4] As with all surgeries, short- and long-term complications can arise. Indepth discussions with your paediatrician and gastroenterologist will have already occurred before considering surgery.

ALLERGY/INTOLERANCE

True food allergies occur in around one in every 20 children (5 per cent of the population) and one in 100 adults (1 per cent of the population). The most common triggers are eggs (hen's), cow's milk, soy, nuts (peanut and tree nuts), wheat and shellfish. The vast majority of food reactions experienced by children are not severe and many grow out of them over time. Usually, by the time they are school age, many children will have grown out of their food reactions; however, there is a small percentage of the population that experience severe reactions such as hives, vomiting, swelling around the nose and mouth, stomach cramping and diarrhoea within half an hour of eating the food. The most severe reaction is known as *anaphylaxis* and involves the respiratory system with symptoms of difficulty breathing, hoarse voice, dizziness or limp, listless children. The foods most likely to cause anaphylaxis are nuts and shellfish. It may become life-threatening if medical help is not available immediately; however, deaths from food allergy are rare in Australia. Allergies must be diagnosed medically through blood tests or skin-prick tests, as self-diagnosis can result in the diet being severely limited in important nutrients which can be very dangerous for growing bodies.

Food *allergies* are often confused with the more common and milder symptoms of food *intolerance*. Allergies involve the immune system and release of histamine causing an allergic reaction when the food is eaten. Intolerances on the other hand are the body's way of telling us that it is unable to process the food properly. A common intolerance in babies and children is the inability to digest large amounts of lactose (the sugar found in milk) or fructose (the sugar found in fruit). Symptoms include bloating, cramping, loose bowel movements and general fussiness when eating.

Some young babies suffer food allergies which may not be immediately obvious. They may develop symptoms such as reflux, eczema or other skin rashes, chronic diarrhoea, and slow or inadequate weight gain (often known as 'failure to thrive'). If you are at all concerned with your baby's feeding or development, see your GP or paediatrician for medical advice.

The incidence of food allergies in children appears to have increased significantly in Australia in the past ten years and we are still at a loss as to why this is. There are many ongoing studies looking into such things as:

- the mother's diet during pregnancy and breastfeeding
- whether or not to delay the introduction of solids in young babies
- the level of processing of our food supply
- skin exposure to allergens such as in almond and peanut oils
- oversanitising our lifestyles leading to an increase in risk.

At present, the recommendations for minimising the risk of developing allergies in children are:

- Do not smoke during pregnancy.
- Do not restrict the maternal diet during pregnancy or breast-feeding.
- If possible breastfeed your child for at least four to six months or use a hydrolysed infant formula for high-risk infants.
- Do not introduce solid food before four months of age.

The introduction of solid foods has been a greatly debated topic for years. We have seen health professionals change their viewpoint or standing on what is the 'correct' time to introduce foods such as infant cereal, cow's milk, egg and fish. Recent studies have suggested that delaying these foods may be associated with an increased risk in developing atopic dermatitis or eczema and may in fact increase the risk in developing an allergy to wheat. Therefore, there is no evidence that dietary restrictions after the age of six months provide a protective effect from allergy development.

POOR HUNGER CYCLE

Every child's appetite is different. You have some who appear to survive on thin air whilst others will eat anything that is not tied down. Some children appear to become hungry almost straight after they have eaten, whereas others can go for hours before they tell you that they need to eat. If your little one is content, and growing happily along their allotted path on their growth chart, then you have nothing to worry about. However, if you have a child with behavioural issues, irritability, minimal weight gain or even weight loss or nutritional inadequacies, then it is important to look at the mealtime routine and more importantly their hunger cycle.

When a child eats, the food is digested and nutrients such as sugars, fats and proteins are absorbed into the bloodstream where they are transported to be used around the body. Sugars rise in the blood which feeds back to the brain which then turns the appetite switch to 'off', essentially saying 'I am full'. This usually lasts for around three hours, at which time the sugars have been used and the body needs refuelling again. The tummy rumbles, you feel light-headed and some may even get the shakes and sweats which is the body's way of telling us to eat. Children, on the other hand, take it a step further. They may become irritable, emotional and unreasonable; however, they just need feeding.

This is a normal cycle, but there is one main difference between adults and children in the window of opportunity in the cycle to feel hungry. Adults will feel the need to eat for about 20 minutes at the end of their cycle, whereas children can have a window of as little as a few minutes. This means they tell you they are hungry so you prepare them their meal only to be told they don't feel like it any more. The missed opportunity is due to the body's starving defence mechanism. Their little bodies start to use stored fuels which suppress their appetite. Understanding this explains why Grandma's theory that skipping afternoon tea in favour of a big nutritious dinner often backfires in spectacular fashion. For these little ones it is all about the timing and being organised to feed them regularly so that they can consume their full complement of nutrients in the day.

Many children are labelled with attention deficit disorder (ADD) or having emotional issues purely due to them not eating regularly enough and adequately fuelling their hunger cycle. A good diet for a child (see Chapter 3) sees carers offering three meals and snacks regularly throughout the day to keep the appetite going. Children need slow release or low GI carbohydrates to ensure slow release of sugars into the bloodstream and adequate protein to maintain their appetite. Think of food as kindling for a fire. Low GI foods are like the logs, burning for a long time to keep the furnace going. High GI foods (think chips, biscuits and lollies) are like paper in the fire, burning very fast to leave nothing. Fuelling with logs makes for a happier furnace. As children grow their hunger cycles become longer and there is more time for them to enjoy their meals.

TONSILS AND ADENOIDS

Many parents are familiar with the angst that infected tonsils can cause. Tonsils and adenoids are made of lymph tissue which is an important part of our body's immune system and helps fight infection. The tonsils and adenoids sit at the back of the mouth and the very back of the nose respectively. They 'guard' our two entrances to the breathing system. Due to their location, they are susceptible to bacterial and viral infections. However, the role that tonsils and adenoids play is small in comparison to other parts of our immune system. This is why they can be safely removed without adversely affecting the way our body handles infections.

The tonsils sit at the very back of the mouth. When the tonsils become enlarged they can look like large balls of tissue jutting out from the sides of the back of the mouth and pushing in towards the uvula (that funny dangly bit that sits at the back of your mouth). Tonsils that are large, red and sore will cause the child pain every time they swallow. Given that we swallow at least 600 times a day (food, drink and saliva), it is not surprising to find that a child with infected tonsils will go off their food. Infected tonsils are often red and inflamed, and may also have a white or yellow discolouration or pus coming from the tonsillar tissue. Not surprisingly, the taste of the stuff oozing from an infected tonsil is not pleasant, and will unpleasantly flavour food and drink. It is not uncommon for some children to reject some foods that were eaten during a tonsil infection. Recurrent bouts of tonsillitis (three to six per year) that seem to recur despite antibiotic assistance will warrant a review with an ear, nose and throat surgeon (ENT surgeon or otolaryngologist) for surveillance and a decision on their removal.

Interestingly enough, infection of the tonsils is not the main reason why tonsils are removed. Enlarged tonsils (also called hypertrophic tonsils), even if they are not infected, can make it very difficult for the child to breathe. Julie recalls one child where the tonsils were so large that they pushed up against both sides of the uvula. The back of the throat could not be seen for the tonsils! Enlarged tonsillar tissue can also make it uncomfortable for the child to have food at the very back of the mouth for chewing because it makes them gag and feel as though they are choking. As a result, these children will choose soft food and will tend to chew food at the front of the mouth, rather than using the more effective chewing surfaces at the back of the mouth. In addition, they may tire quickly during meals, initially coming to the table hungry but rapidly fading as the meal progresses. These children may still be sitting in front of a barely touched plate of food some 30 minutes after the meal started.

A combination of enlarged tonsils and adenoids increases breathing and feeding problems exponentially. The adenoids are lymphatic tissue that sits at the back of the nose, above the back of the throat. Children with enlarged adenoids may be mouth breathers, may dribble, and may be unaware of food around their mouth. Children who Julie has seen who have subsequently had enlarged adenoids confirmed, have also had dark circles and a puffiness under their eyes. Recurrent ear infections are also common in children with enlarged adenoids. This is due to the location of the adenoids and their proximity to the eustachian tube, leading to the middle ear. These children often have difficulty with the sense of smell, may seem permanently congested and their voice may sound as though they have a cold. They may have trouble producing the sounds 'm' and 'n'. At night these children often sleep with their head back, mouth open and often snore. Some children may stop breathing for periods of time during their sleep, which can be quite distressing for parents. They may wake with smelly breath, and be difficult to rouse in the morning. Mealtimes may extend for much longer than 30 minutes.

The effect of severely obstructed breathing, especially during sleep, is a medical concern as it can cause a strain on the heart and the lungs. Recent studies have shown that enlarged tonsils and adenoids have been implicated as the most outstanding risk factor for obstructive sleep apnoea in children.[8] This study further showed a link between enlarged tonsils and adenoids and failure to thrive. Improvements in growth outcomes were noted after surgery to remove the tonsils and adenoids. Growth outcomes for children who had really large adenoids without problems with their tonsils, did not show many changes to their growth patterns after surgery. Julie has used a portable pulse oximeter to measure oxygen saturation in children with grossly enlarged tonsils when they are eating to demonstrate the effect of the obstructive tonsils on their eating and breathing systems. These children need to breathe through their mouth and also put food into that space to be chewed. Imagine putting a sandwich in your scuba mask! Not surprisingly, breathing suffers. Eating becomes hard work and affects the child's ability to take in oxygen. These drops in oxygen during eating increase fatigue. These children can find eating a tiring activity, due to lack of oxygen and lack of stamina.

Where breathing, sleeping and eating are implicated by enlarged tonsils and adenoids, a swift referral to an ENT surgeon is indicated. Whilst children are waiting for surgery, Julie recommends foods that are soft and dissolvable to ensure that they do not use all of their energy in eating. Foods that are nutrient-dense are especially helpful during this time (for example, custard, yoghurt and protein-enriched milk drinks such as Sustagen). Many parents describe a completely different child post-surgery. They commonly describe that they suddenly have a child with energy, a huge appetite and a happy disposition. Recovery from tonsillectomy is associated with reduced appetite, and pain or tenderness on swallowing can be present for up to ten days post-surgery. Keeping fluids up is very important.

CHILDREN WITH BREATHING, HEART OR NEUROLOGICAL CONDITIONS, PREMATURITY AND TUBE-FEEDING

There are some children who have feeding difficulties where you may not immediately expect this to be the case. For example, children who have severe breathing disorders such that their breathing rate is very fast or irregular often have difficulty with feeding. As noted earlier, every time we swallow, we hold our breath momentarily. For a child with breathing difficulties, the body is working first and foremost to ensure that breathing occurs so that oxygen can be pumped around the body and especially to the vital organs. Having to stop this process, even momentarily while feeding, can cause a reduction in circulating oxygen. The child becomes very tired during this process. Consequently, the amount that they eat, and their stamina for feeding, is likely to be reduced. These children may have difficulty with weight gain. In addition, because the swallowing and breathing systems need to work in complete harmony, any disturbance to the breathing system can result in the two systems working out of sync. For some children they may mis-time their breathing and end up with food or fluid 'going down the wrong way'. Infants with conditions such as bronchopulmonary dysplasia (often associated with premature infants) or tracheomalacia (soft and prone to collapsing windpipe) may exhibit these types of feeding difficulties. Usually a medical team at a children's hospital will provide the care and support needed to help the child with their feeding.

Breathing is essential for providing oxygen to the vital organs and the body. In order to get the oxygen to travel around the body, a good pump (i.e. the heart) is required. Conditions that seriously affect heart function (e.g. congenital heart disease) also have an impact on feeding. Some heart disorders may require the lungs to work hard by breathing more rapidly to help provide a continuous source of oxygen to the body. As we have seen above, when the delicate synchrony between breathing and swallowing is disrupted, there can be mis-timing, with an increased risk of food or fluid 'going down the wrong way'. In addition, because the heart and lungs are working so hard just to pump oxygen to the vital organs and the body, fatigue and reduced stamina is also seen. Consequently, these children may tire very quickly during a feed and take only small amounts which makes it difficult for them to gain weight. There is also some evidence to show that these children may also lack a 'hunger drive' and feel full (sated) very quickly. Often, though, this feeling of fullness happens before they have had sufficient food for what they need to thrive and grow.[6]

Pre-term infants are another group that often present with feeding difficulties. It is well-known that premature infants present with breathing difficulties due to immaturity of their lungs. It is probably less well recognised by the community that many premature infants will have difficulty with feeding as well. Infants born prior to 32 weeks of age will be too immature to have developed the sucking skills necessary for feeding. These infants may also have difficulty coordinating breathing, sucking and swallowing. They tire easily. They have weak muscles of the mouth and throat which also makes feeding slow and difficult. They may not wake for feeds or may show little interest in feeds due to immaturity of their awareness of being awake or asleep, hungry or sated. Consequently these infants are often fed via a tube inserted through the nose and running into the stomach. If at all possible, it is important for infants to practise sucking (use a clean finger or pacifier) while nasogastric feeds occur. In this way, the infant learns that activity happening at the mouth (sucking) causes a pleasant and full sensation in the stomach. They will quickly learn that this feeding thing makes their tummy feel pleasantly full. This is something that they wish to happen again and so the cycle of learning about food and hunger and 'feeling full' begins.

Children with congenital conditions such as cerebral palsy, Down syndrome or autism have all been reported to have difficulty with feeding. Some of these children remain stuck on smooth pureed textures. They may also be delayed in developing chewing and cup-drinking skills. This combination of difficulties affects the types of food they eat and consequently their nutritional intake. These children may have difficulty with weight gain. They may also be super-sensitive around the mouth, with poor tolerance to a range of food textures. The strategies described in Chapter 4 have been used successfully with children with congenital conditions; however, the rate of progress is often very, very slow.

Tube-fed infants are another tricky little group. Sometimes tube-feeds are short-term, and other times they can be a more permanent feature of a child's life. Placing a tube down anyone's nose is a fairly confronting activity. It is little wonder that tube-fed infants are wary of people coming towards their little faces! Little ones who are tube-fed may also not have the same oral exploration and mouthing experiences as healthy infants. Little hands edging up towards their mouths may be quickly pulled away by well-meaning adults who are concerned that the child is going to pull the tube out (a fairly common occurrence!). There are often delays in tube-fed infants starting on solids and also progressing through food textures. Lumpy foods can be particularly difficult because this group is often very sensitive in and around the mouth, making gagging and the odd vomit a regular occurrence at mealtimes. This can throw many unsuspecting parents and make them inclined to delay going through that experience again, which unfortunately can make the whole thing continue on for even longer. A team of infant professionals is often on-hand to assist with transitioning these little ones to solids. The group will often consist of a gastroenterologist, paediatrician, paediatric dietitian, and paediatric speech pathologist who specialises in infant feeding. For some infants, eating by mouth is not sufficient to meet all their nutritional needs. For some children a more permanent tube is placed where feeds go directly into the stomach. This means that the nasal tube can be removed. Sometimes it is possible for infants fed via a stomach tube (gastrostomy) to have some small amounts by mouth. The feeding team will advise though, as each child's needs and skills are very different.

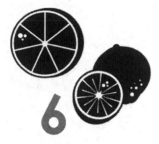

Hiding vegetables in cakes. Is it worth it?

'I used to be able to put carrots and beans on her plate and she would at least try them. Now it doesn't matter how I present them, she just won't have a bar of it. I feel like I spend hours in the kitchen only to have the whole meal rejected. I hear there is a 'vegetable candy floss spray' in the US. Should I use this to disguise the vegetables, or am I doing more damage?'

The skill of hiding things from children has been around for hundreds of years. While hiding healthy food items to get children to consume them without them knowing is nothing new, it seems parents are either losing their touch or children have mastered the art of detection. Some of the most common questions asked are: Firstly whether it is nutritionally worth all the trouble; and secondly is it right to deceive your children or are we setting up bad habits?

IS IT WORTH ALL THE TROUBLE?

Firstly it depends on the age of the child and how adequate their dietary intake is. When babies are trying their first solid foods, they really have no concept of what they are eating. They trust that you are giving them something that they like. As they get older and the variety of foods increases, it is evident that they are starting to develop likes and dislikes. Food aversion often starts when foods become more solid, have stronger flavours, such as broccoli and carrot, and become hard to chew, like meat. This is common between nine and 18 months of age when children start exercising the power of the word 'no'. They have been used to their foods being blended or mashed together, giving a nice smooth consistency and an even, bland taste. Essentially you have hidden the vegetables or meat together with a dominant bland food so that they are easy to swallow with limited chewing required. This is not deception. Mixing foods together ensures that their diets are still balanced and they are getting important nutrients such as protein, iron and fibre which are often lacking when they start turning their nose up at certain foods.

If your child is a good fruit eater but won't touch salad or vegetables with a barge pole, then don't be concerned at this young age as they are probably still getting enough fibre, vitamins and minerals from the fruit. The same applies if they are happy with vegetables but won't eat fruit. When children are young they tend to develop the taste for certain groups of foods before others. Some little ones will munch on a plate of cherry tomatoes and cheese but will avoid all fruits like they were poison. As they get older their tastebuds develop and become accustomed to accepting other food groups. If you are finding that they are turning their nose up at some of the stronger flavours or tough-to-chew foods, then it is better to still mix them together to ensure that their diet is balanced and that they get used to stronger flavours.

A major problem with removing vegetables, salads, fruits or meat from meals is that the diet becomes extremely bland and all the one texture. It is not uncommon to see a toddler's dinner reduced to plain spaghetti with grated cheese or chicken nuggets with baked or fried potato chips. Before their parents very eyes the child's diet has been reduced to half a dozen staple foods which will not provide all the nutrients for growth and development. By adding blended or mashed vegetable into the pasta or mixed into the chicken, it changes the taste and texture and ensures that little ones don't become fussy. The problem with blending all foods together long-term is that they don't develop the chewing processes required for normal development, and this can cause long-term serious complications such as impaired speech development and nutritional deficiencies resulting from fussy eating practices (see Chapter 4). The key is to look at the child's diet as a whole. If they are getting a wide variety of textures, including ones that require chewing such as grainy crackers and whole fruit, then finely grating vegetables into a spaghetti dish or blending vegetables in a sauce is not a problem. The key is challenging and developing their chewing processes and ensuring they obtain enough fibre coming from fruits, vegetables and grains. The most important thing is to provide a balanced diet for the young child. Blending or mashing vegetables and fruits still provides a great source of fibre along with many essential vitamins and minerals. It is important to still offer the fruit and vegetables in their whole or blanched forms alongside their blended or mashed meal, as this helps with familiarity and encourages children to try them. Remember, it can take 10–15 exposures to a new food before a child will even think about trying it, so don't despair if they avoid it like the plague the first few times it is on the plate.

The older child may be difficult to convince and can be more defiant. However, they do have a better understanding of rules and guidelines about foods and mealtimes and you can discuss the benefits of certain foods to the body. For example, 'Protein will help with your muscles and make you run faster'—always a winner with the boys in the family! This is a true test of your negotiation skills. A guideline that works for many families is 'You have to try something first before you tell me you don't like it'. The older child seems a lot less trusting of their parents and it is harder to get them to try something new (see Chapter 8). Again if they are getting a variety of textures from their diet but refuse to eat vegetables, then it is important to 'hide' them somewhere less detectable to ensure they are still consumed.

'DECEPTION'—IS IT APPROPRIATE?

The word 'deception' is very strong and is associated with negative connotations. Disguising healthy food is not deception and is only benefiting the child in the long run. How many times have you heard a mother say their child loved the scones she made only to find that they will never touch them again when they found out they were pumpkin scones? The power of a child's mind is very strong and can influence their perception of taste. Many adults are unwilling to try something that they are unfamiliar with—sushi was not always as popular in Australia as it is today!

Hiding or disguising the flavour or texture of healthy foods in an appropriate dish ensures a balanced diet. However, healthy foods hidden in non-core foods, such as cakes, sweets or deep-fried foods, are *not* advised. Grated vegetables in a meatloaf or rissoles are appropriate, as the vegetable would have been served alongside the dish anyway. However, zucchini grated into chocolate cake or muffins is not doing you or your child a favour in the long run. Firstly, you are sending the wrong message to your child by encouraging them to have a piece of chocolate cake regularly as a meal or snack. Young children become very confused as they get mixed messages and inconsistencies in the food provided to them. They eat Mummy's chocolate cake (with hidden zucchini) which puts a smile on Mum and Dad's faces, only to be told they can't have a different chocolate cake at their friend's party. It looks and tastes like Mum's at home, but they are told it is a party food. This practice also encourages an overly sweet tooth where in fact you are trying to expand on the variety of flavours exposed to your children.

There are a large number of cookbooks on the market 'helping' parents to provide an enticing meal for the young members of the family. Many of the meals require you to be quite artistic with grated vegetables for hair and layered fruits for eyes and nose, and even full movie sets from *Castaway Island* equipped with a green bean drawbridge and olive totem poles. Some children love this concept which has given rise to many food companies producing animal-shaped pastas or branding products with kid-friendly celebrities. There is no problem with this providing the promoted food is a healthy one. The reality is that you can go to an enormous amount of creative trouble only to have the whole meal completely rejected. Children over the age of one should be eating fairly similar meals to the rest of their family with a few minor adjustments for very strong flavours and hard-to-chew foods, especially those foods that require the presence of their two-year molars.

Mixing foods together

Be gentle with your introduction of 'foods mixed together'. Although most adults do not eat this way, children will be more trusting of food that they recognise in the initial stages. They like to be able to point to the carrot, broccoli and potato (even if it is to say 'Yuck!'). Then you can mix it up a bit, providing some meals with vegies sitting ready to be identified on the plate, and other meals where foods are mixed together (e.g. stir-fries or casseroles). A child's view of foods that touch each other can be similar to their perceptions of boy and girl 'germs'. Over time children come to appreciate foods mixed together. They will then be more open to mixing foods together or consuming foods with sauces, dressings or additions.

Most Australians today enjoy a multicultural diet including curries, stir-fries and pasta dishes all requiring ingredients to be mixed together in some form of sauce. For most people this is a more palatable way of eating and sauces help with chewing and swallowing foods. Dry chewy meats and lukewarm blanched vegetables are actually very difficult for children to chew and swallow, often taking in excess of an hour to finish. By this time the dinner has gone cold and become even less palatable. Familiarity and ease breed success. Realistically, children should sit for a maximum of 30 minutes at the table.

For the fussy child:

- Start with a smaller than usual serve.
- Make sure that all foods on the plate are still warm.
- Cut foods into bite–sized pieces.
- Provide dipping sauces to moisten and lubricate the meal.

HOW AND WHAT TO HIDE

The three most difficult food groups to get children to eat are:

1. Fruits and vegetables
2. Protein (meat, chicken, fish and eggs)
3. Milk.

Fruits and vegetables (excellent sources of vitamins, minerals and fibre)

The first thing that most people think of when it comes to an alternative to fruit and vegetables is juice. The average home has some form of juicing machine and some families consume excessive amounts of fruit and vegetable juices thinking they are healthy. Fruit juices are not recommended for children as they are high in kilojoules (natural sugar is still sugar and contains kilojoules that the body has to burn off), lacking in fibre (the pith and the skins contain fibre and usually the best bits end up in the bin after the juicer is cleaned), and may lack vitamins B and C found in fresh fruit.

Use the juice in fruit cakes or in some breakfast cereals like bircher muesli, or better still use the whole fruit either finely grated or blended as a topping in yoghurt, over low-fat frozen yoghurt or blended into a summer fruit smoothie. Blending fruit with low-fat frozen yoghurt and refreezing makes great kids' ice-creams for summer. There are not many ice-creams available that contain fibre and vitamins! Grated or stewed fruit can be added to muffins, pancakes or pikelets. Finely sliced banana or apple can be layered on pizza bases for a dessert pizza.

Roasted vegetables can be blended and strained into a basic tomato sauce to use with spaghetti, pasta and meatballs or as a pizza base covering. This will provide vitamins, minerals and fibre without your little one having to chew down on any vegetable. Vegetables such as pumpkin, corn, zucchini, carrot and potato can be creamed and added to savoury muffins, pies, quiches or baked into scones, scrolls or homemade breads. These vegetables are also very easy to add to minced meat, chicken or fish and rolled into nuggets, rissoles or savoury cakes. The vegetables not only provide some bulk and great health benefits but also add subtle flavour to encourage a developing palate. Most times children object to fruits being too slimy and vegetables being too chewy and stringy. The above solutions (and more in recipes below) minimise the slimy and stringy textures of foods.

Potato and pumpkin pancakes

150 g potato
150 g pumpkin
1 egg
½ cup self-raising flour
Olive oil for frying

Peel and roughly chop potato and pumpkin. Place in food processor and blend until smooth. Place in bowl, pressing down to remove excess water. Whisk egg and add to mix with flour. Mix until like a paste. Heat a pan with oil over medium heat. Place tablespoonfuls of mixture into pan. Lightly fry each side until golden.

Kids can help with the food processor.

Zucchini slice

1 onion, finely chopped
Bacon
2 large zucchini (approx. 300 g), grated
1 medium carrot, grated
1 cup grated cheese
1 cup self-raising flour
½ cup oil
5 eggs, lightly beaten
Salt and pepper to taste

Microwave or lightly fry onion and bacon for 1 minute. Combine zucchini, carrot, cheese, bacon and onion in a large bowl. Sift in flour, add oil and eggs. Season with salt and pepper, and mix to combine. Pour into well-greased pie or quiche dish. Bake in a preheated oven at 180°C for 40 minutes.

Note: If top starts to brown, cover with foil to continue cooking.

 Easy to freeze.

Kids can crack the eggs.

Mini carrot cupcakes

125 ml olive oil or 125 g margarine
1¾ cups wholemeal flour
½ cup soft brown sugar
1 cup sultanas
2 eggs, beaten
2 tablespoons honey
2 small or 1 large carrot, peeled and grated
Juice and zest of 1 orange

In a large bowl, rub olive oil or margarine and flour together until it resembles breadcrumbs. Add sugar and sultanas, and stir to combine. Add egg and honey, and stir. Add carrot and orange juice and rind, and stir. Place even amounts into muffin tin or patty cases. Bake in a preheated oven at 180°C for 15 minutes or until just golden. Makes 12 cupcakes.

Easy to freeze.

Kids can help by mixing in between each step and arranging and placing mix into patty pan cases.

Roast vegetable tomato sauce

500 g ripe tomatoes
1 small butternut pumpkin, peeled
1 carrot, peeled
1 zucchini
2 cups chicken stock
1 clove of garlic
½ onion, finely chopped
400 g tinned tomatoes

Chop tomatoes, pumpkin, carrot and zucchini and place on a baking tray lined with baking paper. Roast in preheated moderate oven for 30 minutes. Place baked vegetables in food processor and blend with 1 cup of stock. Strain liquid through sieve. Place liquid in saucepan and add garlic, onion, tinned tomatoes and remaining stock. Simmer gently for 30 minutes. Sauce can be stored in containers and frozen.

Easy to freeze.

Zucchini and walnut loaf

3 eggs
1½ cups brown sugar
1 cup oil
1 cup walnut pieces ━━E
1½ cups grated zucchini
1½ cups wholemeal self-raising flour
1½ cups plain flour

Grease a 15 x 25 cm loaf tin and line with baking paper. In a large bowl, beat eggs, sugar and oil until creamy. Stir in walnuts, zucchini and sifted flours. Spread evenly in tin and bake for 1½ hours in a preheated moderate oven.

━━E Leave out walnuts for children under 2 years or if there is a nut allergy concern.

━━ Easy to freeze.

Apple and sultana muffins

2 cups self-raising flour
1½ teaspoons ground cinnamon
½ cup brown sugar, lightly packed
1 cup milk
90 g butter or margarine
1 egg, beaten
2 Granny Smith apples, peeled and grated
½ cup sultanas

Sift flour and cinnamon into a large bowl. Add sugar. Add milk, butter or margarine, egg, grated apple and sultanas. Mix with spoon until combined (don't overmix). Spoon evenly into muffin tins. Use patty pan cases in the large trays; the muffins travel better this way in lunchboxes. Bake in a preheated oven at 180°C for 20 minutes until golden brown (tops will spring back on touching). Cool on wire rack. Makes 12 large or 24 mini muffins.

Easy to freeze.

Kids can help crack egg, mix and spoon into muffin tins.

Pumpkin scones

1 tablespoon butter or margarine
2 tablespoons sugar
Pinch of nutmeg
1 egg, beaten
1½ cups mashed pumpkin
2–2½ cups self-raising flour

In a large bowl, cream butter, sugar and nutmeg, then add beaten egg and pumpkin. Gradually stir in flour till a dough forms. Roll out to 2 cm thickness and cut into circles using a cookie cutter or glass. Place scones close together on a lightly greased baking tray. Bake in a preheated oven at 220°C for 15 to 20 minutes or until golden.

 Children can help roll out dough and love using different-shaped cookie cutters.

Easy to freeze.

Fresh fruit icy poles

400 g peeled chopped fruit such as pineapple or melon
1 punnet strawberries

Blend pineapple or melon and spoon in as first layer of ice block. Blend strawberries and spoon in as second layer. Place plastic ends or ice-block sticks in each segment and freeze. Makes six.

Kids can use the blender if supervised.

Meat and chicken (excellent sources of protein, iron and zinc)

The reason why children reject meat and chicken is not usually the taste but the texture. You need a lot of power in your jaw and teeth to adequately chew and break down meat into a nice paste to be swallowed. Most babies enjoy the taste of meats and chicken blended or finely minced into their meals; however, when it comes to chunks it requires a lot more effort. To compound this, children are usually given these sorts of meals at night when they are tired. What usually happens is they chew and chew and chew the meat until it becomes so dry or has the texture of a piece of chewing gum. Essentially their saliva dries up and they find it nearly impossible to swallow the piece so they spit it out. This can turn a relaxed dinner table into a battleground which is stressful for everyone. Before children develop their molars they do find it easier to consume softer proteins such as fish, baked beans and eggs which are all high in protein, iron and zinc and are a great substitute for the tougher, drier meats. Red meat is still an essential part of the diet but you may have more success in presenting it in an easier form to chew.

The food processor is an essential machine in any kitchen and is handy to mince red meats and chicken for meals such as meatloaf, homemade sausage rolls or rissoles. You can also process some vegetables such as zucchini, carrot and sweet corn in with the meat for added fibre and vitamins. White fish and chicken can be processed and rolled into healthy fish cakes and chicken bites. If you are still finding that the protein part of the meal is being rejected, then using legumes is a fantastic alternative and can go undetected. All legumes are high in protein, iron and fibre whilst supplying slow release carbohydrates for energy. Hommus made from chickpeas can be used as a dip or spread on a sandwich or pizza base as an alternative to meat or chicken. Baked beans, refried beans or any tinned legumes again contain an excellent source of protein and iron which is an alternative for meat. Red lentils can be added to soups and sauces and once cooked they are virtually undetectable and are very easy to digest whilst supplying a similar set of nutrients as red meat.

Winter meatloaf

1 onion, peeled and chopped
1 tablespoon olive oil
1 teaspoon crushed garlic
100 g lean bacon, chopped
400 g veal mince
300 g pork mince
2 tablespoons tomato sauce
1 tablespoon Worcestershire sauce
1 egg
2 cups grated wholemeal bread
Topping
20 g Parmesan cheese, grated or shaved
½ cup extra breadcrumbs

Place all ingredients except topping into a food processor and process until mixed thoroughly. Line a loaf tin with baking paper. Press meat mix firmly into tin. For topping, mix breadcrumbs and cheese and spread over top. Bake in a preheated 180°C oven for 1 hour or until golden. Serve with tomato sauce (see Roast vegetable tomato sauce on p. 157) and vegetables.

Kids can help with the processor and pressing meat into loaf tin.
Easy to freeze.

Falafels

400 g can chickpeas
¼ onion, finely chopped
½ teaspoon cumin powder
½ teaspoon ground coriander
1 clove garlic
1 tablespoon flour
Olive or canola oil for frying

Place all ingredients except oil in food processor and blend till smooth. Roll tablespoon amounts into balls. Shallow-fry in olive oil or canola oil until golden. Drain on paper towel. Serve immediately.

Kids can help mix and roll into balls.

Hommus pizza

4 tablespoons hommus
4 tablespoons pizza sauce (or tomato paste)
4 mini pizza bases
80 g haloumi cheese cut into 12 slices
8 cherry tomatoes, thinly sliced

Spread 1 tablespoon hommus and 1 tablespoon pizza sauce on each base. In a pan, lightly dry-fry the haloumi cheese on both sides. Arrange sliced tomatoes and haloumi cheese on pizza. Place under hot grill for a few minutes until base is golden at the edge. Serve with salad.

Kids love dressing the pizzas. They can spread the hommus and tomato paste using the back of a large spoon. They can also arrange the tomato segments and place the cheese on the top.

Beef rissoles

400 g lean mince
1 egg
1 onion, peeled and grated
½ cup finely grated vegetable (carrot and zucchini work well)
½ cup breadcrumbs
1 tablespoon tomato sauce
1 teaspoon Worcestershire sauce

Mix all ingredients in a bowl. Separate into 4 lots. Roll into balls and flatten out to about 12 cm diameter. Place on baking tray. Bake in a preheated moderate oven for 25–35 minutes or until cooked through. Serve with multigrain roll and salad or vegetables. Use tomato or soy sauce drizzled over rissoles if needed.

 Easy to freeze.
Kids can assemble their own hamburger.

Fish cakes

425 g can tuna or salmon (or white fish for bland flavour)
1 onion
2 sticks of celery
1 carrot
garlic, ginger to taste
1 tablespoon oil for frying
1 tablespoon flour
salt and pepper to taste
2 potatoes, cooked and mashed
1 egg, lightly beaten
breadcrumbs for coating

Drain tuna or salmon. Heat oil in pan. Finely chop onion, celery, carrot, garlic and ginger and fry for 5 minutes. Transfer vegetables to a bowl and add flour, salt, pepper, and drained tuna or salmon. Add potatoes and beaten egg. Cool. Shape patties then cover in breadcrumbs. Makes approximately 15 patties.

Easy to freeze.
Kids can help roll the patties.

Golden chicken bites

300 g chicken breast fillet
1 carrot, peeled and chopped
½ cup corn kernels
1 zucchini, chopped
½ cup tasty cheese
½ tablespoon soy sauce
1 tablespoon cornflour

In a food processor, process chicken until smooth, then transfer to bowl. Process carrot, corn kernels and zucchini, and transfer to bowl. Add cheese, soy sauce and cornflour. Mix all ingredients well. Roll tablespoonfuls into balls and place on a baking tray lined with baking paper. Bake in a preheated oven at 180°C for 30–40 minutes until golden.

Easy to freeze.

Milk

Very few babies completely reject breast milk or formula unless there is a problem. However, a number of little ones stop drinking milk when they start solid foods. There doesn't seem to be any pathological reason why they do this, some just prefer food. Others drop milk like a hot potato when it is offered in a cup rather than the beloved bottle.

Transitioning over from bottle to cup by your child's first birthday will reduce the likelihood of this happening.

Milk provides a great source of energy, protein and the important mineral calcium. Some adults also have definite ideas on the ways in which they will take their milk. Some are big drinkers of smoothies, milkshakes and milk coffee, whereas others can go for weeks without any milk. There is no problem providing the diet is balanced and other high-calcium foods are included. Yoghurt, cheese, custard, white sauces and calcium-fortified soy products can be used as a substitute.

The aim for children is to include three calcium-rich dairy foods each day. The following are equal in the amount of calcium they supply to the diet:

- 1 cup of milk or calcium-fortified soy milk equals
- 40 g cheese equals
- 200 g yoghurt

For example, your child's daily intake can be made up of two 100 ml tubs of yoghurt plus cheese on their sandwich and sprinkled on their dinner and 200 ml milk. Use milk in a white sauce in a meal of macaroni cheese or lasagne, or made into a smoothie and frozen into ice blocks. This diet is balanced for calcium without taking one sip of milk.

Some children actually don't like the taste of plain milk and are happy to drink milkshakes or flavoured milks. This is not a problem providing you control the amount of flavouring that is added. A small teaspoon of Milo or some frozen vanilla yoghurt or low-fat vanilla ice-cream blended with the milk is a healthy option to encourage children to drink milk.

Cheese cannelloni

200 g butternut pumpkin, peeled, cooked and mashed
250 g smooth ricotta
100 g creamed cottage cheese
⅓ cup grated cheese
3 egg yolks
1 teaspoon garlic
1 teaspoon nutmeg
10 cannelloni tubes
400 ml tomato sauce (see Roast vegetable tomato sauce on p. 157)

Place all ingredients (except tubes and tomato sauce) in bowl and mix well until thoroughly combined. Fill each tube with mixture. Use half the sauce to cover the base of an ovenproof dish (approximately 20 cm x 25 cm). Arrange the filled tubes in a single layer on the sauce. Cover the tubes with remaining sauce. Bake in a preheated oven at 200°C for 30–35 minutes.

 Kids can help fill the tubes.
Easy to freeze.

Banana smoothie

150 ml milk
2 large spoonfuls of low-fat vanilla ice-cream or frozen yoghurt
1 banana, peeled and chopped
1 tablespoon honey

Place all ingredients into a jug. Use a handheld blender to blend well until smooth. Serve with straw. Makes 2 drinks.

Baked custard

1 cup milk
1 tablespoon caster sugar
1 teaspoon vanilla essence
1 egg yolk

Mix milk, sugar and vanilla in a bowl. Beat egg yolk, add to bowl and stir in. Pour into 4 ramekin dishes. Place dishes into a baking dish containing 2 cups of water. Bake in a preheated moderate oven for 15–20 minutes or until just set.

Strawberry frozen yoghurt

1 cup strawberry yoghurt or low-fat frozen yoghurt
6 fresh strawberries

Place yoghurt and strawberries in a blender and blend till smooth. Place in individual ice-cream moulds. Freeze.

WHEN TO DIG YOUR HEELS IN

Disguising healthy foods in the early years is fine, and blending some fruits and vegetables into foods that kids will eat is a healthy option. However, there will come a time when you must stand strong or seek further help. If your older child is not having variety and is refusing to try anything new, then there is a risk of a long-term unbalanced diet and nutritional deficiencies. Seek help from a chewing and swallowing specialist and possibly a psychologist to help your child overcome the fear of trying and eating some foods. Don't just treat the symptom, treat the cause of the problem.

7

'The rules of engagement'—Rules at mealtimes

The family sits down to dinner. All of the children have washed their hands and faces and are sitting smiling as dinner is laid in front of them. There is carrot, cucumber, baby spinach leaves, alfalfa sprouts, tomatoes, and some tender strips of marinated lamb. The children gaze adoringly at their mother and thank her for all of her hard work in the kitchen, exclaiming how wonderful dinner looks. They proceed to sit up straight and tall, and use their knife and fork to devour every last morsel. The 3-year-old politely asks for more. Dinner is over in 15 minutes and the cherubs are happily scooting off to have their bath. This is not reality. Welcome to planet 'In your dreams'!

Ask any parent and dinnertime is resoundingly voted the most dreaded meal of the day. Everyone has their horror story of a nasty childhood mealtime experience or ritual. Personal experience as a youngster of an introduction to steak and kidney pie and its dramatic reappearance some two mouthfuls later has dulled only a little over time. People now in their 60s recall being forced to sit at the table till all was eaten, regardless of whether the sitting took 20 minutes or two hours. In the latter case, fat was congealed on meat that had been cooked in lard and vegetables were stone cold; hardly a visually appealing or appetising meal. Women in their 30s and 40s recall being dished up the remnants of their uneaten dinner for breakfast the following day. Many a dining room wall has resounded with the call of 'If you don't eat your peas/carrots/broccoli/[insert the vegetable or other food item], you won't have any dessert.' Parents have also been known to use guilt to entice their offspring to eat. Surely children must realise the amount of time it has taken to prepare the wholesome nutritious meal placed before them; just as surely they will eat it all unquestioningly.

It is likely many of these personal horror stories and experiences have today's parents trying to figure out and handle the 'rules of eating'. Eager not to have their own children remind them of the time they were forced to eat some ghastly concoction, many parents have thrown their hands up in despair in the hope that their children will fall into step, and eat as members of civilised society. Unfortunately, the 'let's hope for the best' method does not seem to be yielding high stock returns. Children require some guidance and boundaries for mealtimes.

However, it is not just children who need mealtime rules. Parents also need to understand and stick to the rules of engagement. They should be clear about their household rules so that children know what to expect. Rules that keep changing are very hard to anticipate and will only increase the anxiety levels of all concerned. This chapter provides information about some of the things that commonly go wrong at mealtimes and ways of troubleshooting them.

TIMING IS EVERYTHING—THE 'PERFECT TIME' FOR MEALS

My 4-year-old tells me he is hungry so I start preparing his meal. By the time I put it in front of him, he says he doesn't want it and proceeds to have a tantrum.

Meal timing is everything, especially with young children's appetites. Probably the main cause of food refusal at night, as described in the quote above, is a delayed dinnertime. Most adults have experienced their appetite 'switching off', especially when they are busy or pre-occupied. When our bodies are starting to run low on blood sugar, we get a few warning signs such as light-headedness, the shakes, memory loss and a rumbling stomach. Children experience this as well but the symptoms are more intense; children happily playing together can quickly turn on each other and the cries of 'You're not my friend' and 'I hate you can' start filtering over to the oblivious parent. This is usually a sign of a drop in blood sugar. Parents constantly report that arguing children can often be quelled by giving them something to eat. This 'haywire' behaviour is the body's way of telling us that we need to eat.

There is a window of opportunity for most adults to eat within about 20 minutes of these signs before our urge for food decreases. If we don't eat within this time, there is a built-in safety mechanism where a different form of fuel is used to keep our bodies running. This process will suppress the appetite at the same time. This is why you can feel unbelievably hungry one minute but by the time you get around to eating your appetite has gone. This is exactly what happens to children except that their window is around seven minutes, which doesn't leave parents a lot of time for preparation. The key is to make sure children are fed approximately every 2½–3 hours. So if they have breakfast at 6 a.m., morning tea at 9 a.m., lunch at 12 p.m. and afternoon tea at 2.30 p.m, then they may need dinner at 5–5.30 p.m. Trying to push your little one out to 6–6.30 p.m. will only end in disaster as their desire for food decreases. If you are having no success with the dinner meal, try bringing the timing forward to see if they are hungrier.

Eating regularly is not only important to keep our appetites going, it ensures that we consume a healthy diet. Another common mistake is missing a meal in the hope that your child will have a bigger appetite when they next eat. Parents will often avoid giving afternoon tea thinking it is 'spoiling their child's appetite for dinner'. Often the reverse happens and the child becomes less interested in the dinner meal. Afternoon tea at 2.30 p.m. will be completely burnt and used for energy by 5–5.30 p.m. when they are ready to eat again. If meals or snacks are regularly missed, your little one may not be obtaining all the necessary vitamins, minerals and energy that they require for the day. The Dietitians Association of Australia recommends that people eat three meals and snacks and do not skip meals, especially breakfast.

MORE ABOUT DINNER MEALS

The perfect picture that every parent is looking for is one big happy family sitting around the dinner table happily eating together and enjoying everything on their plate. This is a rarity when very young children are involved. The first stumbling block is the time. In most households one or both parents work till at least 5–6 p.m. which can make it difficult to get everyone to sit around the dinner table at a reasonable hour. Young children tend to be very tired by 4.30–5 p.m. and also very hungry. If they are made to wait until 6 p.m. and onwards to eat when Mum or Dad get home, then it can be a disaster. Children often get overtired and their appetite can switch off, which leaves them cranky and unwilling to eat anything. This is often confused with defiance and fussy eating where in fact they have just been pushed to 'hold on' for too long.

The current recommendations for family dining are that families eat together without the distraction of television or video games. This enables the family to interact and parents to lead by example even if they are simply munching on some salad or vegetables whilst their younger children eat their dinner. With over-stretched working parents, many have interpreted this to mean that children should eat with them at 7.30 p.m. It is possible, however, to have younger children fed at an appropriate time for them and still meet the 'family mealtime' recommendations. Any adults or siblings who *are* home early can sit at the table whilst the youngest member of the family has their early dinner. It is important that Junior is not left alone at the table for meals. When Mum or Dad come home from work and are ready for their meal at the adult time-slot, children can rejoin the table. While Mum and Dad are eating a full meal, Junior can have a healthy snack (e.g. a yoghurt). Children who are not hungry can still join the table and tell their parents about their day while Mum or Dad eats. Family communication is preserved. The important experience of watching adult role models eat is retained, and yet children also manage to eat at a time appropriate for *their* little systems.

The reason why children cope better with an early dinner has much to do with proximity to bedtime. As adults who might go to sleep at 9.30 p.m., we are unlikely to be interested in a roast dinner with all the trimmings, no matter how nicely presented, at 8.30 p.m. or even 9 p.m. Children who are in bed at 6.30 p.m. are unlikely to be interested in dinner at 6 p.m. They have often been up for around 12 hours and have been playing hard. They are tired. Their parents are tired from chasing after them, playing with them and then cleaning up or putting in a full day at the office. In our experience, even through into the school years, dinner offered as early as 4.30 p.m. or 5 p.m. will be eaten very well. A healthy snack may hit the spot in that half hour to an hour before bed, but the big work of digesting a full meal should be over well before children go to sleep.

As children get older they are more capable of stretching out their mealtimes to eat with Mum and Dad a bit later. The timing for family meals tends to be more successful on the weekend when everyone can eat together. There are many benefits to eating together such as seeing other people eat different types of food and observing 'civilised rituals' such as using cutlery. Children also learn dinner-table manners, for example, waiting until everyone is finished before leaving the table. This teaches patience and helps little ones get to know the rules. This is particularly helpful for those attending day care or even children about to start school—one big set of rules!

THE TIMING OF OTHER MEALS AND SNACKS

We've mentioned above that on average we should be looking to eat about five times a day. For the household who wakes early, breakfast may be on the table as early as 6.30 a.m. For other families, breakfast may not be until 7.30 or 8 a.m. The child who starts with breakfast at 6.30 a.m. will likely be ravenous and ready for more food by 9 a.m., while the late-waking child may be ready closer to 10 a.m. Little wonder that childcare centres can struggle to find a 'good time' to serve children their meals. Some little tykes will have well and truly missed their hunger cycle, while for others it will be perfect for them to devour their food with gusto (see Chapter 5 for more information on hunger cycles). Table 18 below provides a rough guide to anticipated mealtimes for early- and late-waking households.

Table 18: **Mealtimes depend on waking times**

Meal	Early-waking household—wakes at 6 a.m.	Late-waking household—wakes at 7.30 a.m.
Breakfast	6.30 a.m.	8 a.m.
Morning tea	9 to 9.30 a.m.	10.30 to 11 a.m.
Lunch	11.30 a.m. to 12 noon	12.30 to 1.00 p.m.
Afternoon tea	2.30 to 3 p.m.	3.30 to 4 p.m.
Dinner	5 p.m.	6 to 6.30 p.m.

EATING MEALS REGULARLY 'AT THE TABLE' VS 'GRAZING'

Children should be encouraged to sit down for meals, preferably at a table. Sitting at mealtimes has a couple of important functions. First of all it means that they can focus their attention on what they are doing, namely eating. Eating at the table reduces the risk of choking. Toddlers especially who come and take bits of food from communal areas and walk around with it in their hands and mouth do have an increased risk of stumbling and possibly choking on a piece that gets lodged in their throat. Choking on food is a very real threat, particularly to under-fives. Sitting is better for digestion and it also helps parents to know what the child has eaten. Sitting in a highchair at the table can encourage little ones to be more experimental with their food when they see what everyone else is eating. Getting a little one into a routine early can often reduce the problems with fussiness later on, as they become comfortable and familiar with the mealtime process.

Sitting for even 5–10-minute periods also helps children learn to keep their bodies still. As they grow older, sitting still is required on the mat at childcare or kinder and for longer periods of time as they enter school. Sitting down to a meal also helps a child to learn that sitting means the meal has started and standing up and walking away means that it has ended.

Three meals a day plus snacks in between is a healthy way to feed your child. In fact it is a healthy way for all of us to eat. Eating in this manner keeps the metabolism going and ensures adequate nutrition through small frequent meals. Children's stomachs are very small and so they fill up and empty quickly. Eating regular meals and planned snacks is preferred to 'grazing' which many children get in the habit of doing. When a child is constantly eating, they are not filling up and registering 'fullness' or satiety. Not being able to recognise the signs of feeling full is the first step to overeating. Children who regularly graze develop a constant hunger and are always looking for their next meal.

Children need to learn to regulate their appetite. Apart from excessive kilojoules, grazing can also become unhealthy due to the types of foods that are constantly eaten. Common grazing foods include crackers, juice, milk, biscuits and bread. Many of these foods don't require a great deal of chewing. Interestingly, research shows us that the process of chewing is very important to our desire to keep eating. Foods that can be consumed in less than five minutes (e.g. soups, soft foods or dissolvable foods like crisps or chips) do not help the brain or gut to register feeling full. Meals that take between 15 and 20 minutes to chew and swallow help the body to recognise the signs of fullness. After this time the brain registers that the taste of food is not as pleasant as it had been at the beginning of a meal and we lose our desire to keep eating.[1]

'SIT STILL, STOP FIDGETING AND DON'T PLAY WITH YOUR FOOD!'

Whew! You may as well ask a cow to stop producing milk! Little people have short attention spans. In general, girls have longer attention spans than boys; and an attention span of about five to ten minutes would not be unrealistic with most children. In fact the adult attention span is widely quoted as about 20 minutes. This information needs to be applied to mealtimes. Grey hair, crow's feet, defiant cranky children and permanent scowl lines are the only things to be gained from having a child sit at the table for an hour or more. What your child has not eaten in the first 15 minutes is unlikely to be eaten. This may also be finely tuned with the body's response to feelings of fullness, which also kicks in after around 15 to 20 minutes, as described above. Aim to have mealtimes served and cleared away within 30 minutes.

We want our children to pay attention and to sit still. Stop for a moment and think about where your child generally sits to eat. A little table and chairs, designed for little people, is a terrific spot for toddlers. Sitting at the kitchen table often means sitting on a grown-up chair. Little feet do not touch the ground on a grown-up chair and so little feet will swing. Those of us who are 'vertically challenged' will recognise that sitting on a barstool can be difficult if there is no bar to rest your feet on. You have to wriggle back from time to time to keep your balance and be comfortable. Swinging your legs also helps your body to know where it is in space. The same thing happens with children. Ways to alleviate this issue at a dining table include using a chair where there is a foot support or providing a stool for children to place their feet on, touching a solid surface, which helps to 'ground' them. Layering up phone books can provide a cheap alternative to a footstool.

Children are often roused on for 'playing with their food' and for using their fingers for eating. Early feeding experiences are both messy and time-consuming. Loading up the spoon, and ensuring that the fully laden spoon makes it all the way to the mouth without depositing too much on the floor or in the lap, is a tricky business for a learner driver. It is often not until the child is about three-and-a-half that they can independently load the spoon and deliver it to the mouth without too much spillage. Table 19 below provides other key 'cutlery milestones'.

Cutlery skills use a combination of large and small muscles of the arms and hands. Fine motor skills, like holding a pencil or a fork, come first from having strength and stability in the arm muscles (large muscles). You need good stability in the big muscles to allow the fine movements further down the chain to take place. Like a tree, the trunk also needs to be strong and children need good trunk support to be able to sit up at a table. Strong back muscles, and also arm and hand muscles, come from regular physical activity. It is important for children to run and climb to make these big muscle groups strong. The big muscles can then act as a ballast and allow the child to fine-tune the use of their smaller muscles. If you are concerned about your child's walking or climbing skills, a paediatric physiotherapist may offer assistance. If you have any concerns regarding your child's cutlery use or fine motor skills, a paediatric occupational therapist should be considered.

Table 19: **The ages of independent cutlery use**[2,3]

Age	Independent feeding skill
6–9 months 9–13 months 13–15 months	Uses a cup with help. Finger feeds soft foods. Holds cup with both hands; takes a few sips without help. Dips spoon in food; moves spoon to mouth but is messy and food often spills.
15 months 15–18 months 18–24 months	Emerging self-feeding skills—scoops food with spoon and feeds self. Uses a straw. Wants to be independent and feed self.
2 years 2½ years	Drinks from an open cup (no lids) without spilling contents. Feeds self entire meal when food is cut up.
3 years 3½ years Almost 4 years	Pours liquid into glass with some spilling. Uses spoon to feed self with limited spilling. Puts dry cereal and milk in a bowl without spilling. Holds and uses fork to stab food and bring it to the mouth.
4½ years	Uses knife to spread soft food.
5 years	Uses knife for cutting.

Why do children play with their food? Let's sort the fact from fiction. In many cases children are not 'playing', they are enquiring with their fingers as to the textures of the food so that it gives them an idea of what it will feel like in their mouth. Eating with their fingers helps children to develop a textural awareness of food. Of course, we need to introduce our children to the civilised use of cutlery. However, even for school-aged children, unless you are dining with the Queen, it is okay to allow some latitude for some finger feeding. Pick your battles. If your child is happy to eat that piece of steamed carrot using their fingers and insistence on the fork is going to leave the carrot on the plate, go with the fingers. Hands can be washed after dinner. An astute parent will be able to sort out when their child is overly fingering food and is in fact looking for a parental reaction. In this situation, children should be redirected to use their cutlery, or to finish and leave the table.

Mess is to be expected when children eat. Even with a family of primary school children, sweeping under the table after dinner is a regular occurrence. For younger children, a bath *after* dinner means that children can eat without being concerned about keeping their clothes in pristine condition during the meal. They can be bathed, hop into clean pyjamas and then have a story before going to bed. This kind of routine also helps children to anticipate what will happen next. Children who have a regular routine tend to be calmer.

'FINISH YOUR PLATE'

One of the most common questions asked by parents is 'How much does my child actually need?' The answer is that children tend to know themselves. We can all remember our parents telling us that we could not leave the table until everything was eaten, which often included the cold lump of spinach! This ensured that there was no wastage of food and that we would grow up big and strong. Unfortunately, this approach promotes force-feeding and an inability to self-regulate appetite. Children, unlike many adults, know when they have had enough. Forcing them to eat more is teaching them to push beyond this trigger and eat more than they need. Most adults will register fullness between 25 and 40 minutes after they have eaten, whereas some children can have this 'I'm full' feedback mechanism within about ten minutes. This is due to a couple of reasons. Firstly, children have small stomach capacities. Secondly, protein foods such as meat, chicken, fish, cheese and eggs stay in their stomach longer than other types of food and help them to register that they are full.

From a very early age your child will either be a 'foodie' (one who loves food) or a 'sparrow' (one who eats the bare minimum to survive). It is quite amazing that both types of eaters grow into perfectly normal healthy adults. You will quickly become familiar with your child's desired serving size. Give your child too little and they will demand and look for more; however, provide too much and they may be overwhelmed to the point where they reject the whole meal. If you are worried by the lack of foods being eaten by your child, have a check-up with your GP or see an accredited practising dietitian to analyse your child's intake for nutritional adequacy.

There is not a parent alive who has not implored their child to finish their meal. Unfortunately, research shows that children respond by eating *less* when they are nagged or 'encouraged' to eat, than if left to their own devices. Not only do children tend to eat less when we pressure them to eat food, but they also develop negative attitudes towards the foods they are pressured to eat.[4] In fact, apart from liking the food less, children also complain more about the food when pressured to eat. As shown by the stories from adults in their 30s, 40s and older, these negative effects follow us into adulthood. What about rewarding children with a treat for eating their vegetables? Unfortunately, offering a reward for eating also seems to result in a reduced liking of the food. Although tempting, bribery with dessert is not the answer.

So how does a parent implement the 'no nag, but secretly I want you to eat your dinner' tactical manoeuvre? First things first, remember to begin with a reasonable portion size. Many is the child who has sat at Grandma's table looking at a mountain of food fit for a grown-up and desperately tried to get to the bottom of the asparagus so that they can escape from the table. So, starting first with a reasonable portion size, the following can be used as a general guide:

- If they have eaten *half their meal* and say they are full, ask if they have room for one last mouthful and then they are done.

This approach lets children know that you respect that they are filling up and also allows them to listen to their body.

- If they have eaten somewhere between *a quarter and a half of their meal,* which may not seem to be enough, then halve what is left and remove one half from the plate. This is far less daunting and easier to conquer. If they still refuse, they may be in a food jag associated with growth spurts or have missed their hunger cycle (see Chapter 5). Do not be alarmed, request a final mouthful and monitor general appetite over the next few days.

- If they say they are full and *haven't had one spoonful,* then either they have had too much for a snack before the meal or they are exercising their right to reject the meal, which drives most parents around the twist. Without fuss remove the plate, letting your child know that nothing else is available for dinner. If they decide they want to attempt dinner again, serve up half the plate, remembering to give it a quick reheat if it has gone cold.

Sometimes distractions—such as older kids playing, a television on in another room, or parents interacting away from the child—can be enough to break the child's concentration, causing them to stop eating and tell you they are full. What they really want to do is watch the TV or play with their siblings. The problem here is that their desire to interact with someone or something temporarily switches off their appetite, which returns a short time later with vengeance. The key to success is a quiet, comfortable place to eat that is free from distractions. However, children left alone to eat at the table without any company are likely to lose interest pretty quickly. Ensure that an adult sits with children during meals. Remember also that children's appetites fluctuate depending on their age, their wellness and the energy expended during the day. When feeding children, dramatic changes in appetite are the norm.

In short, provide an age-appropriate amount of food at a time when they are going to be most receptive to eating. As noted above, this is not 20 minutes prior to them going to bed. Teach them how to try new foods, and, yes, you can use non-food rewards here. Chapter 4 provides details for coaching children on how to try new foods. Next, you set your expectations and communicate these: for example, 'I expect you to take a bite of everything on your plate. After that you can decide how much to eat, but remember there is nothing more after this until breakfast.' Then play poker and bluff, bluff, bluff. Talk about the day, things you are looking forward to, the child's favourite book, anything in fact other than the food on the plate. If you are really stuck for ideas, there is a great pack called 'Table Topics' that is a box full of conversation starters. This group has also produced a kids' version with gems such as 'If you could choose a new toothpaste flavour, what would it be?', 'What would you love to invent?' and 'What would you do if you were invisible for a day?' Other ideas to take the focus off the food at mealtimes include games like 'Celebrity Heads', 'I Spy', or for little ones 'I hear with my little ear…' Allow the meal to progress for no longer than about 30 minutes. At about that magic 30 minute mark, regardless of what food is left on the plate, ask your child whether their tummy is full. If the answer is no, remind them that there will not be anything else to eat till breakfast, and so if they are still hungry now would be a good time to eat. If they indicate that they are full, then clear the plates and move on with your evening routine.

PARENTAL PARANOIA ABOUT FOOD INTAKE

Our reasons for wanting our children to eat healthy foods heartily are well-intentioned. However, from our children's perspective, it is another opportunity for parents to tell them what to do. In this situation though, the child holds the ultimate decision on whether or not to eat. They exert control over their environment and also over their parents.[4] It is helpful to remember that food is not the only area that children make a fuss about. At some stage every child will become an ironing board when inserted into their car seat, making it nearly impossible to do up the seatbelt. Other children will run and scream at the sight of the sunscreen bottle. However, parents deal with these situations and children learn to wear a seatbelt, a hat and sunscreen. You won't hear a parent say, 'My little Angela just simply refuses to wear a seatbelt.' So why is it that we struggle so much with food?

Warmth, food and shelter are some of our most basic physiological needs. When we are hungry or thirsty, our bodies are unbalanced. This imbalance shows itself as tantrums, whingeing and other problem behaviours, being 'fragile' and anxious or even feeling sick or uncomfortable. Humans are wired to ensure that we eat and that our offspring eat. As parents, we become anxious when our children do not eat. Many parents who pressure their children to eat are concerned that their children are not eating enough to meet their nutritional needs.[3] We forget, though, that children will often eat very little when they are sick. They may go for a few days with relatively little food and we will rationalise that they are not eating because of their illness.

Some parents assume that night-time waking is due to hunger. Being sleep-deprived makes for cranky parents. Assuming that a big dinner will solve the problem, parents begin to pressure their child to eat all their dinner. Many children do still wake at night, but it may be because they are cold, or have had a bad dream, or need to go to the toilet. Do not assume that hunger is the reason or even plant the hunger thought in your child's mind if they wake during the night. Work through other possibilities, such as being cold or needing to go to the toilet. For children who truly have not eaten sufficiently, and complain that they are hungry, offer a glass of water. This sends a clear message for midnight marauders that there is nothing special on offer when the rest of the world is asleep. Be consistent with this approach and you will find that children learn very quickly not to expect a drink of milk or a biscuit in the middle of the night. Given the choice of a glass of water or sleep, sleep wins out.

Today's parents are also more informed about food choices and food nutrition. They strive to meet the daily quotas for fruit and vegetable intake, and may feel that poor intake is a reflection of their parenting skills.[5] Public health messages are well-intentioned. It is our job to provide appropriate foods to allow children to meet their nutritional needs, but it is the child's role to decide how much to eat. Children's intake can fluctuate noticeably over the course of a week, unlike an adult who has stopped growing. Monitoring children's intake over a week rather than daily may help more parents to relax.

BRIBING WITH SWEETS—'EVERYDAY' FOODS AND 'SOMETIMES' FOODS

We have all been down the bribery and corruption path, but will it help our children to choose healthy foods in the long run? The answer is no. It is even in the way we phrase it that is problematic. We put the emphasis on the ice-cream and couple it with a big smile. In fact we are saying that if you gulp down the tasteless vegetables on your plate, you can be rewarded with some fabulous ice-cream. Rewind and Mum could say: 'Did you know that your zucchini and carrots are like ambulances to help your body to build new skin for where you grazed your knee? When you've finished sending in your ambulances, can we play a game together?' This gives a reason for the food choice and something positive to look forward to after the meal.

Rewarding with 'sometimes' foods creates more problems later, when children will only eat vegetables if followed by ice-cream. These non-core foods are truly 'treats' and are not needed in the diet. It is important to start at a very early age to distinguish between 'everyday' foods and 'sometimes' food. Provide 'everyday' foods within reach of children in pantries, fridges or on tables where they can see and access them. 'Sometimes' foods (treats or party foods) should not be readily visible to cloud children's choices. Highly refined foods with excess sugar, fat and salt should not make their way into young children's diets on a regular basis and should not be used to bribe them to eat the healthy option first. Australian children are being taught the concepts of healthy eating at an early age with many preschools, kindergartens and primary schools running nutrition programmes for their students. It's up to us as parents to reinforce this at home.

For parents, the key is to explain why some foods are more important to eat than others. Talking about vegetables and salad in terms of 'fighter pilots' in your system, and milk and yoghurt to help make your hair shiny is a better way to encourage children to eat. Older children will understand more about the roles different foods play, such as meat providing iron or calcium-rich dairy foods for bone strength. There are more ideas for different ways of explaining the roles of different foods to children in Chapter 8, 'Surviving the older child'. It is okay to occasionally reward eating a challenging meal or trying something new with a non-food reward. Rewarding children with a movie or playing a game together is better than using 'sometimes or party food' as the reward.

WHY DO WE GO DOWN THE SWEET FOOD PATH IN THE FIRST PLACE?

Food is linked to comfort. This is a link established at birth to ensure that we survive. As noted earlier, breast milk is sweet and the process of feeding releases endorphins in the infant that are very pleasurable. The infant learns that feeding feels good, and so they continue to feed and look for food. During the phase of typical food fussiness we need to understand that children are rewiring their circuits and learning about food flavours and textures for themselves. There is increased communication and a sense of emerging independence. An ability to control their environment and say 'No!' is part of their evolution.

Somewhere deep down, parents know that food can be used as a great motivator. Animal shows at theme parks confirm that tricks can be taught when followed by a food reward. Parents attempt the same process with their children using sweets and treats as rewards. This process only elevates the status of the sweet or treats. It does nothing to increase the liking of the 'problem food'.

To increase acceptance of a food you must have repeated exposures to it. However, the moment we try to control the intake of the food, any gains made from repeated exposures are lost. In short, we have to play the best poker face and game of bluff that we can. By showing no reaction to whether a food is eaten or not reduces the 'power' of the food. In order to do this though, there are some guidelines that need to be set in place.

PARENTS—REALISTIC EXPECTATIONS, PLEASE

All children are different; whether it is height, eye colour, personality or, you guessed it, eating habits. Your first-born may have eaten everything in front of them whereas number two may pick like a sparrow. The bottom line is that if they are growing well along all health charts, then they are fine and you may need to lower your expectations. Some children simply survive on less food or are very happy with repetition. If they are consuming a balanced diet with plenty of variety, they may just be a child who is not that inquisitive, or responsive to change. Issues arise when dietary intake becomes so limited that it is unbalanced or children are failing to thrive. In cases such as these, it is important to seek professional help to ensure that your little ones are given the healthiest start in life.

TRYING A NEW FOOD—PUTTING IT INTO PRACTICE AT A MEALTIME

You have gathered your courage and decided to introduce a new vegetable to the dinner table. It is probably one that you have introduced to your child using the strategies outlined in Chapter 4. Harry was happy to eat one round of steamed carrot and so now you are going to put steamed carrot onto his plate for dinner. Keep your expectations realistic. Put just one small piece of carrot on his plate and remind him that it is 'easy-peasy' because he's done it before. It is achievable and he will feel successful because he can manage it. By all means ask if he would like more, and then let him choose how much more without making comment about how much he chooses. However, if the answer is 'no', then praise him for having the piece he did and remind him that his body will thank him for it. Parents, remember that he's doing it for his own health, not for you. If he says 'no' and you try and load another three pieces onto his plate, he will feel as though he has been tricked and will be less likely to do what you ask the next time. He's done what you asked, and by forcing more you are changing the rules and punishing him. Day two is when you increase the amount a little bit more, and so it goes day by day with gradual increases. This process may take a couple of weeks to get it to an ideal amount. Similarly, a child with a very restricted diet (e.g. the 'white food child') will not change their diet in 24 hours or even a couple of weeks. It will take patience and consistent yet gradual changes to significantly alter this child's food variety. Strategies for establishing new habits are detailed in Chapter 8, 'Surviving the older child'.

PARENTS—WATCH WHAT YOU SAY IN FRONT OF YOUR CHILDREN

Monitor carefully what you say in front of your children. Whisper the word 'chocolate' from the kitchen pantry and see how many little faces appear to get a good grasp on your children's hearing range. Like it or not, even when we think our children are not listening to boring grown-up conversations, they are taking it in like a background radio. Whenever you start a sentence with 'My child doesn't eat . . .', you are reinforcing and telling the child that they don't eat that food. They simply follow your direction. Use language that encourages them to try food. Train yourself to repeat the message that 'Jenny is good at *trying* foods'. From the child's perspective you are providing an achievable goal; trying a food is different to being expected to eat a plateful of food. Learning to try foods is important. They didn't know they liked cupcakes till they tried them.

BUILDING CHILDREN'S CONFIDENCE AND HELPING THEM LEARN TO MAKE DECISIONS ABOUT FOOD

As parents, one of our roles is to help children to be confident to try foods. Another parental role is to also be comfortable to accept that children may not want more *just now*. Remember that children are growing and changing. It takes many of us years to become accustomed to the bitter taste of coffee, but once hooked many can't start the day without it. Respecting your child's decision to say no from time to time is an early decision-making skill that can empower your child and build their confidence. Parents usually despair at this point and howl that if left to their own devices their children would eat chips, chocolate and soft drink all day—this is true. However, children can only eat those foods if you purchase them and have them in the house. Your role is to provide food that you want your child to eat. Their job is to listen to their bodies and work out how much they need. It is part of a supervised and growing independence.

One research group developed a set of rules for 2–3-year-olds presented with a buffet of healthy food from which to choose.[6] The rules, as follows, make some good sense: 'I choose what I want, in the order

I want'; 'I can take several foods at the same time'; 'Before taking more food, I eat everything I have chosen'; 'I do not take the same food more than three times'. In each case one serving spoon counted for a serve of food. With these rules children did not gorge themselves on a single food. In fact, the researchers found that children chose the same food twice in 10 per cent of cases. In only one per cent of cases was a food chosen three times. Notice that the rules empower the child to choose.

RULES FOR HOME AND FOR VISITING FRIENDS AND FAMILY

We all have our own ways of doing things. We have most control in our own home. Consistent rules at home mean that children know what behaviour is expected. When we move out of home we are transitioning behaviours to a new environment. Whether it is a trip to the grandparents or a lunchtime barbecue with friends, changing the scenery alters mealtime dynamics for children in one of two directions. They will either surprise you by happily eating foods that you would not have dreamed they would touch, or they will misbehave because there is nothing they like. Some parents 'rescue' their children by bringing a small esky of the child's favourite foods so that they do not have to try new foods. The rescue package also means that parents will not have to deal with their child's performance if there is nothing the child likes.

Let's look at the worst possible scenario. You arrive at Aunty Gertrude's and your child takes one look at the lunch spread and shrieks that there is nothing she likes. You have not brought any rescue food. They will choose the least offensive item and nibble on it, or they will refuse to eat at all. If they refuse to eat, will they die? No. Will they get sick? No. Will they become irritable and cranky? Possibly. It is this last one, that as parents, we want to avoid. We have an expectation of a lovely lunch with adult conversation and the last thing we want is our child whingeing and moaning that they are hungry and that there's nothing to eat. It's time to be a parent.

If your child has been taught to try new foods you can take them by the hand, remind them that they know how to try a new food and ask them to choose one. Better that they choose the food, because you have a higher chance of success. Then ask them what the steps are for trying a new food and praise each step they move through. It is then their choice whether they have more or even try some different food. If, for one day, they choose to have a small meal or just a taste, they will not die or become malnourished. We also need to grow a thick skin to possible disapproving looks or comments from other adults. You may wish to tell them that this is the way you try new things at home, that they won't die, and then move on with your lunch—don't you or other adults make a fuss! Some adults may need a more direct approach—politely remind them that it is none of their business.

Some children use a mealtime outing to audition for their spot at the National Institute of Dramatic Arts (NIDA). They love being the centre of attention. Food is the perfect ammunition to get the fireworks started. These children also need to be reminded that they have been taught how to try new foods. If they refuse, they need to be reminded that this is their choice. No further attention. Any whingeing and whining needs to be redirected to a reminder that they are choosing not to eat. A stint on the 'thinking stair or spot' and other behavioural techniques are required. Although it is uncomfortable and may take you away from adult company for up to 20 minutes while you deal with it, the child learns the consequence. They will not be likely to try it again in a hurry.

Forward planning can help a lot when eating away from home. If you know that a good family friend always invites you over for lunch at 12 noon, but doesn't start preparing it till 1 p.m. with the meal not on the table till 2 p.m., you need to take action. Feed your children before you go. Then they can snack at the lunch table. Adults can wait; children can't and shouldn't be expected to. Similarly, if the food on offer really is exceptionally gourmet, it is reasonable to ask for a plain roll, a piece of fruit or a simple sandwich for your child.

Help your child by preparing them in advance. We are going over to Georgie's house and it is likely there will be some new food to try. We'll have a look together and see what we can find. Be wary of adult comments such as 'I've made spaghetti because everyone likes spaghetti!' Spaghetti at Kate's house is likely to be different to spaghetti at Julie's house and different again in each street of every suburb. Same name, different beast. Children may love Mum's spaghetti, but can be very disappointed when somebody else's spaghetti doesn't taste exactly the same. Children need information that the same name can mean it will taste different; the important message is to try it. Julie's children have happily informed her mother-in-law that her mashed potato tastes heaps better than Mum's! As adults we have to accept that children are naturally honest and do not develop the skills to provide censored feedback until they are adults themselves. As hard as it can be after you've slaved for an hour in the kitchen, sometimes adults need to grow a thick skin and let negative feedback roll off their backs.

PLAY-DATES

It is extremely hard to police everything that goes on when someone else is caring for your child. Hopefully, if you have befriended people with the same ideals as you, the job won't be so hard; however, there are occasions when your little one will come home with a mouthful of chewing gum gloating that he has consumed the better part of 1 litre of cola. If it is a one-off occasion then there is not a lot you can do about it. If it is a regular play-date, it is worthwhile just talking to the parent or carer. You could explain that you would prefer to send some food for everyone to enjoy, and could they leave the gum and soft drink for when your little one has gone home. It is hard feeling like the 'diet police' but your young child will very quickly become accustomed to these sweet-tasting foods and demand them regularly. If you send a platter of food, include things like dips (such as hommus or avocado) with grainy crackers, vegetable sticks, chopped fresh fruit and cubes of cheese. These foods when mixed with some of the refined foods will dilute the sugar. Try not to cave in to the demands of a 4-year-old.

For the older child you can explain the differences between healthy foods and treats. A good strategy is to ask them to have their fresh fruit first before they have any party foods (see also 'Bribing with sweets: Everyday foods and sometimes foods' (p. 184)). For the fizzy drinks issue, try to pull your dentist onboard and get him or her to explain what sugary foods and drinks do to their teeth. These are not shock tactics. It's just that children tend listen to those in authority (especially those wearing white coats) over their parents. If your child does have a sugary drink or juice, just ask them to have a glass of water afterwards.

GRANDPARENTS, GRANDPARENTS, GRANDPARENTS

Something happens between the time your parents are relieved of their 'parenting duties' and take up the role of the treat-giving grandparent. They now feel it is their duty to never say no to your children and provide a never-ending supply of sweet and party foods. Essentially, they are Santa Claus moonlighting as your mother and father! They are only too happy to let their grandkids purchase and devour $5 worth of mixed sweets half an hour before dinner regardless of the fact that their offspring are dietitians or dentists!

There is also another take on today's generation of grandparents. In this age where both parents work, some grandparents have become the main caregiver for their grandchildren. Often grandparenting style will affect success at mealtimes. Some grandparents are young at heart and free-spirited, while others are more stately and can be sticklers for manners and rules. The biggest key is balance, commonsense and good communication. When grandparents have returned to the role of primary carer, we need to clearly communicate how we want them to deal with our children's meals and mealtime behaviour. Consistency will help the children know what is expected by the grown-ups in their lives and the odd treat will not kill them.

SPECIAL OCCASIONS

Birthdays, parties, etc.

Birthdays, parties, sporting functions, etc. are a time for celebration. These things usually happen half a dozen times a year and are not worth worrying about. If you are hosting any of these functions or asked to bring a platter, you can still offer some healthy options to outweigh the 'kilo of sugar' provided per child. The key is to provide some foods containing protein as these delay the stomach emptying and slow down the release of sugar into the bloodstream. Yes, we have all seen children running around screaming excitedly at parties after they have grazed at the party food table. Did you know that the jury is still out as to whether the offending elements are colours, additives, excessive sugar or just pure excitement? In any event, having a bit of protein to line the stomach cannot hurt. Protein foods are meat, chicken, fish, eggs, cheese, milk, yoghurt, nuts and legumes. Some handy party foods containing protein are meat pies, sausage rolls, sausages, cheese bites, hommus or Mexican bean dip, sandwiches with cheese, peanut butter or meat, and chicken or fish balls, bites or nuggets. Naturally, if you made these yourself, you can control the amount of fat, salt and additives that go into them; however, if you need to purchase them, just read the label and choose the healthiest option.

Restaurants

We recall one mum nearly in tears telling us that one of her dreams was to be able to take the family out to dinner at a restaurant. A child who has learned to try new foods at home, and knows that 'I have to try a bite and then choose whether to eat more', will be well-prepared for a trip to a restaurant. A bit like our earlier discussions about realistic expectations, there are even steps we can put in place to help young children gradually get used to eating in public.

Toddlers have a short attention span. Dinner with a toddler in a highchair at a swanky restaurant at 6 p.m. has 'train wreck' written all over it. You have to crawl before you can walk. Your first public restaurant–type outing might be for a cup of coffee for yourself and a milkshake for your child. If you wish to order food, look for something that is already prepared. Drinks come quickly at restaurants. Food that has to be cooked will often take a minimum of 15 minutes, by which time your child is climbing on the table. Experience some success. Encourage your child to sit and drink their drink while you drink your drink. Praise them for sitting well and then leave! For those first few visits keep it for just you and your child. Inviting another adult will divert your attention and may make the visit longer than your child can tolerate.

For proper restaurant dinners as children get older, you can ask for drinks to be held back and served with the meal so that children do not fill up on their drinks leaving no room for the food that has finally arrived. Research your restaurant well and have a good idea of how long meals take for preparation. See if the location is such that one adult can take the children for a walk while they are waiting for their meal. A local restaurant may use butcher's paper as a tablecloth and provide a collection of crayons to keep little fingers busy while they wait for their meal. Stickers and colouring-in books can also while away the time.

Kate has some excellent suggestions for ordering from the menu. Children may like to order their favourites, but should be encouraged to have a taste or a try of a food from Mum or Dad's plate. Also look for entrée serves for children to keep portion sizes to realistic expectations. The Cicheros have a fun family rule. On the first Friday of each month Julie does not cook and the family goes out for dinner. This has become a lovely family tradition with the children providing lots of ideas for different places to eat or styles of food to try. The aim is to go to a new restaurant or try a new food each time.

Surviving the older child

Waiting for the first mouthful of solids is closely matched in anticipation to the utterance of your child's first word. You spend the first year of your child's life waiting for them to learn to talk. By the time they hit four years of age and every sentence they utter starts with 'Why?' you begin to wonder what all the excitement was about. Life with a toddler is challenging because they are still learning the language. Communications come in a brevity akin to text messages, and miscommunications are common. 'Ohh, *that* apple, the red one that looks remarkably like a tomato (mutter, mutter).' Older children are unique because they *can* communicate. Of course this brings its own frustrations as they provide you with every adjective known to man that conveys 'yuck' when their meals are not to their liking.

As we become parents of older children, we begin to realise that fussiness is not restricted to the littlies of the family. Most parents' angst comes from frustration that their older children are not eating adult meals and, therefore, everyone in the family is still restricted to eating 'kiddy' style meals. Many fussy toddlers can grow into fussy 8-year-olds if the problem is not dealt with when they are young. Big kids who are unwilling to move beyond plain pasta or Vegemite sandwiches run a greater risk of developing nutritional deficiencies such as low iron stores, zinc deficiency or inadequate calcium deposition in their bones.

The worst-case scenario is stunted growth due to the fact that the body has not had enough fuel and building blocks for basic growth processes. Now before you become paranoid that your youngster is doing permanent damage, write down what they are eating for a few days. This is known as a diet history and gives you an idea of what your child eats in a 24 hour period. What it also shows is that some days they consume everything they need (and sometimes more), whereas other days appear to be a little 'light-on'. Over the course of a week you will probably find that everything averages out, and they are consuming a healthy diet. (Refer to Chapter 3, 'What is a good diet?' to compare their diet history to the average requirements.)

There are two main reasons why it is very important to keep encouraging your older children to increase the variety in their diet. Firstly, their requirements increase quite dramatically after the age of nine, and it is very hard to satisfy all the nutritional requirements when the diet is limited in choice. Secondly, it is a time when the land of restaurant dining, playing at other people's houses, camps and 'the sleep-over' starts to emerge. For many parents, what their child eats is a 'parenting barometer'. Just how good are their parenting skills if their children don't eat certain fruits and vegies? Some parents are particularly frustrated, because they have tried their best to ensure their offspring eat fruit and vegies. If this is you, you are not alone! This chapter will provide information to help parents to negotiate with their older children and the best ways of teaching their children to make good choices for themselves.

INCREASED ENERGY AND NUTRIENT REQUIREMENTS

As children get older, the main nutrients that are needed in much higher amounts are protein, fibre, iron, zinc and calcium.

Protein

Protein is used for growth and repair, with the main sources coming from meat, chicken, fish, egg, legumes, and dairy or soy foods. The minimum protein requirement for a 1–3-year-old is 14 g, which is satisfied by a 30 g piece of meat and a glass of milk. How do you work out what 30 g looks like? 100 g is about the size of your palm, so 30 g is about one-third of the size of your palm. Protein requirements increase again by the time they reach nine years; this time the requirement is 20–40 g. This can be satisfied using 60 g of meat, a glass of milk, a tub of yoghurt and 30 g of tuna or chicken on their sandwich.

Fibre

Fibre, or roughage, comes from wholemeal flours, wholegrain cereals and breads, fruits and vegetables. Children aged 1–3 years need 14 g of fibre per day, whereas a 9-year-old needs an extra 10 g per day. A piece of fruit contains about 3–4 g of fibre and a piece of multigrain bread contains 2–3 g, so you can see how important it is to encourage little ones to progress on to wholegrain breads and cereals and fruit with the skin.

Iron and Zinc

Iron and zinc are two of the most important minerals for growing children. Zinc assists wound healing, helps maintain the body's sense of taste and smell, and is needed for DNA synthesis. Zinc also supports normal growth and development during childhood and adolescence. Iron helps transport oxygen around the body in the blood supply. Both are important minerals involved in the immune system. They are essential for fighting the green nose gremlins that come home from kindergarten and school!

The richest sources of iron and zinc are red meat, fish (e.g. tuna, salmon), chicken, egg, legumes, fortified cereals and dark green leafy vegetables. The estimated average requirement of iron and zinc for a 1-year-old is 3–4 mg per day compared with 5–6 mg per day for a

9-year-old. A 100 g serve of red meat can supply around 4 mg of iron, and a serve of iron-fortified cereal will supply around 3 mg of iron. The requirement is not hard to achieve for both age groups providing they eat the foods! If your children are not big meat, chicken or fish eaters, then you need to find alternatives. (See 'What to do when important foods are avoided' in Chapter 3.)

Calcium

Calcium is extremely important in the early growing years for healthy teeth and bones. The calcium requirements for a 1-year-old are 500 mg compared with more than 1000 mg at age nine. A glass of milk, small tub of yoghurt or a piece of cheese can provide around 300 mg of calcium each. Most children love milk but it is important to continue to provide variety. Yoghurt has the added advantage of healthy bacteria for the gut, and cheese provides a good source of calcium that can be added to sandwiches or used as a snack. If your child doesn't like milky products, calcium-fortified soy or using milk to make creamy sauces provide alternatives that can bump up the calcium.

Table 20 below is a quick guide to show the increased energy and nutrient requirements, as your child gets older.

Table 20: **Serves of food groups required per day**

Age	Daily requirements
1–3 years	5 glasses of fluid 1 serve fruit + 1 serve vegetables or salad ½ serve meat, fish or chicken 2 serves full-cream milk, yoghurt or cheese
4–8 years	6 glasses fluid 1 serve fruit + 2 serves vegetables or salad ½ serve meat, chicken or fish 2 serves reduced-fat milk, yoghurt or cheese

Age	Daily requirements
9–13 years	8 glasses fluid 2 serves fruit + 3 serves vegetables or salad 1 serve meat, chicken or fish 2 serves reduced-fat milk, yoghurt or cheese
14–18 years	9 glasses fluid 2 serves fruit + 5 serves vegetables or salad 1 serve meat, chicken or fish 3 serves reduced-fat milk, yoghurt or cheese

What is a serve? Use the examples provided in Table 21 below. (More information is available from the National Health and Medical Research Council of Australia publication 'Dietary guidelines for children and adolescents in Australia' or at http://www.nhmrc.gov.au/PUBLICATIONS/synopses/dietsyn.htm).

Table 21: **Examples of one serve**

Food group	One serve equals
Fruit	1 medium sized fruit (apple, banana or orange) 2 small sized fruit (apricot, plum, kiwi fruit) 20 grapes 1 cup canned fruit Dried fruit—4 apricots, 1½ tablespoons sultanas
Vegetable/salad	1 medium potato $1/2$ cup cooked vegetables 1 cup lettuce/salad
Meat, chicken, fish, egg (Remember that 100 g is about the size of the palm of your hand)	65–100 g cooked meat, chicken 80–120 g cooked fish 2 small eggs ⅓ cup cooked legumes (dried peas, beans, lentils)

Food group	One serve equals
Milk, yoghurt, cheese	1 cup milk (250 ml) 40 g cheese (2 slices) 200 g carton yoghurt
Cereals, breads	2 slices of bread 1 cup of porridge or breakfast cereal flakes 1 medium bread roll 1 cup of cooked rice, pasta or noodles

SUSTAINED ENERGY REQUIREMENTS

Older children need more menu planning, especially once they go to school. The main difference is that children attending kindergarten, preschool and school have to learn to wait and eat at designated mealtimes. The young toddler learning the pattern of mealtimes is usually hungry every two to three hours. Mum or Dad can chop up a bit of fruit or provide a quick savoury cracker to fill a hungry gap between meals. This is where things start to unravel for the fussy older child. If they haven't eaten enough food, or enough of the *right* foods at the designated mealtime (e.g. breakfast), then they have to wait until their first break at school, which might be three to four hours later. This is extremely difficult on the child (and their teacher) because as blood sugar levels are falling so is their behaviour. Some children are not disruptive or naughty they are simply hungry and don't know how to contain these actions and feelings. Other children just simply slip off their perch and fall asleep. The key is to provide foods that sustain their appetites.

Appetite-sustaining foods are also known as low Glycaemic Index (low GI) foods, with the energy from them released slowly to last over a few hours. Naturally occurring long-lasting foods are wholegrain breads, cereals and crackers, most fruit with the skin, pasta, milk and yoghurt. You can also make a meal last longer by adding a protein-rich food such as meat, chicken, fish, egg, cheese, peanuts and legumes such as baked beans. For example, a Vegemite and cheese sandwich will sustain a child's appetite for longer than a plain Vegemite sandwich. A few plain crackers will last longer if you put some peanut butter on them, or provide them with hommus or avocado and cream cheese dip. Even the humble healthy piece of fruit can last longer in little ones' tummies with the simple addition of yoghurt to the snack. If your child is a 'plain food' eater and picks at dinner only to come back an hour later saying 'I'm hungry', look at including some protein, such as an egg or half a cup of baked beans or even some cheese on toast.

FAVOURITES

By the time your child is around five years of age they have definite ideas on which meals are their favourites. These are the ones requested most nights of the week. It is okay to have a favourite meal, just not every night. You know yourself when you go to a regular restaurant that you can fall into the habit of ordering your favourite meal. This is partly because you love it and partly because you don't want to order something only to discover that it wasn't as nice as you thought it might be. These same thought processes go through a child's head: 'What if I don't like it?' or 'What happens if it tastes yucky?' So they opt for safety and stick with the known meal. Use their favourite meal in a positive way, explaining that they didn't know what it was like before they tried it. Having a few favourite meals picked by members of the whole family is a great way to negotiate a new meal onto a menu. Explain that everyone in the family has to try each other's pick. This is also a great first lesson in learning the art of compromise.

CHILDREN'S ACTIVITY LEVELS INFLUENCE APPETITE

Children's energy needs vary. Energy requirements will vary depending on the activity levels of your child. Physical activity is important for bone and muscle growth, fitness, posture and flexibility, in addition to a wide range of other skills (e.g. balance, hand–eye coordination used during throwing and catching a ball). Very young children are constantly on the move, often slowing down only when they need a sleep. Children aged 5–18 years of age should be aiming for about 60 minutes of physical activity every day. This will likely happen in bursts, but when it is all added together should account for at least an hour of activity, if not more. A combination of 'moderate activities' and 'vigorous activities' is recommended by the Australian Government Department of Health and Ageing. Some ideas for moderate and vigorous exercise are included in the table below.

Table 22: **Types of exercise**

Type of exercise/activity	Examples
Light physical activity	Walking, playing outside, playing on playground equipment, skipping, hopping, jumping, hide and seek
Moderate physical activity— equal in intensity to a brisk walk	Game of tag/tiggy, bike riding, dancing, riding scooter or skateboard, trampolining, skipping with a rope, gymnastics, handball, martial arts
Vigorous physical activity— these activities make children 'huff and puff'	Ballet, running, swimming laps, soccer, football, tennis, basketball, netball

A Queensland Healthy Kids Survey (2006) found that the most popular physical activities for 6-year-olds are playing, skipping and trampolining or playing on playground equipment. Bike riding was a popular activity for most ages. Common sports across all age groups were soccer and athletics. Younger children were most interested in handball whilst touch football was popular amongst older children.

There will also be increased energy requirements during growth spurts. Parents of teenage boys are well-renowned for their stories of their boys eating them 'out of house and home'. During puberty, boys triple their muscle mass, whereas at this time, girls double their muscle mass. Parents need to remember that for the entire period of growth (i.e. birth to 18 years) appetite and energy needs will vary. Adults' energy needs are fairly constant, with exceptions for exercise and illness. It can be easy to forget that children are *not* little adults, but growing individuals. Parents should *expect* change in appetite and be flexible enough to cope with these changes to avoid problems.

WHY OLDER CHILDREN CAN BE FUSSY

The advantage of having an older child with fussy food habits is that you can talk and reason with them. Sit down one afternoon and find out why they don't 'like meat' or 'hate fruit'. You will probably find it comes down to something simple, like it is too hard to chew or feels too slimy. Often children have tried something along the way and they have hit a particularly chewy chop or overripe rockmelon that has left a lasting bad impression. They then start to avoid all similar foods for fear of coming across the offending article. In the meantime, they become so reliant on their 'regulars', or safe foods, that they are too scared to try other foods. A beef chop may be avoided for its toughness; however, you could explain that beef in a rissole or a meatloaf is exactly the same but so much softer. Ask your older child to help with food preparation to show them how it is made. This practice often helps to alleviate the fear of trying something, because there are no surprises.

Maturing tastebuds

It is worth noting that tastebuds do change as children get older. Younger children have many more tastebuds than adults do, so foods that taste relatively innocuous to adults can give young children the sensation of fireworks. Remember the funny screwed-up faces your baby made when you gave them some bland rice cereal for the first time? Research shows that children with high taste acuity (e.g. 'super-tasters') are more often associated with fussy eating.[1]

Apart from our tastebuds, we also use our sense of smell to taste the flavour in food. Remembering that food tastes blander when you have a cold is proof enough of this concept. Chewing food is important for detecting flavour. Chewing produces saliva, this mixes with the food and helps the tastebuds to recognise flavours. The jaw-closing action in chewing also sends pockets of flavour-laden air up the back of the mouth to the back of the nose (cribriform plate) where our smell detectors are located. So, a heightened sense of smell will also enhance the flavour of a food. If you have a child who can smell Grandma's perfume long after she has left the car and your own sense of smell can detect nothing, your child may be blessed, or cursed, with a superior nose. Taste and smell are both important for detecting the flavour of your food.

You may find that you have struggled for years trying to get your 7-year-old to eat a certain food, such as chicken, only to find that they come home from Gran's place announcing that they love chicken skewers with peanut sauce. Don't take offence to this. It was probably just that their tastebuds were ready. Note, though, that when children stick to bland foods for too long, they will experience a more intense taste from *normal* foods. Providing them with more variety, little and often, is critical. Continuing to encourage children to try new tastes will do wonders for helping them to develop a tolerant and flexible taste palate.

Defiance

It is a parent's dream to have strong-willed, driven, motivated and confident children—just not every night at the dinner table! Sometimes defiance has to be reined in. There may come a point when fussy eating and a failure to try anything new comes down to pure defiance. Some older children get into such a rut that they actually don't know how to ask for help. Parents and carers need to step up and set some ground rules before fussy eating gets out of hand.

Fight the battles you need to win! If your child eats red meat and fish, don't worry if they don't touch chicken. If they love strawberries, pear and grapes but hate all rockmelon, pineapple and watermelon, it is not a problem. They are still getting an excellent source of vitamins and fibre from the fruits they love and they will eventually try other fruits as they get older—just take a look at your likes and dislikes as a child. The main concern for your older fussy child is if they are eliminating whole food groups such as all fruit, all dairy or all proteins.

Another very important fact to remember is that children will not willingly starve themselves. Sending your children away from the table hungry because they have not had their way is not child abuse. It is merely stating that '*This is dinner*, if they choose not to eat then they will feel hungry'. They soon learn that there is a set of rules around mealtimes. Yes, there are some very defiant children out there who will yell and scream for hours whilst others will take themselves to bed without a word. With some positive, reassuring (firm) words, your children will begin to follow the rules; just like cleaning their teeth or going to bed at a certain time. Think how you would react if they flatly refused to go to bed or clean their teeth. Apply this reaction when they refuse to touch their food. The main thing to establish when setting guidelines is consistency. There is no point being firm and sticking to your guns one night only to turn around and give in the next. Children will learn nothing from this and you will take an enormous step backwards.

Parental sabotage

Despite their best intentions, parents, without thinking, can sabotage their children's eating habits. In full hearing range of their children, parents will calmly announce that 'Mary is a very fussy eater!' or 'Mary doesn't eat any fruit' or 'That really looks lovely, but no, Mary won't even touch that quiche'. Mary is being told what she does and doesn't do. Now she may not eat fruit, but if Mum and Dad keep telling her that, then that is what she comes to expect of herself. A psychologist colleague pointed out that given an opportunity to try fruit, her first thought is 'I'm the kid who doesn't eat fruit. If I try this and maybe even *like* it, will Mum and Dad still give me attention?' Parents, if you choose to seek professional assistance regarding your child's eating habits, it may be worthwhile making that first appointment just by yourself. Give yourself the opportunity to say what it is you want to say about your child and their eating habits, but without them as an audience to confirm the things that really push your buttons. As you try to establish some new habits with your child, make a conscious effort to provide positive messages for them to drink into their psyche. 'Mary always gives new things a try. She's a very good eater…' It's time to start reprogramming!

'Because I said so, that's why'

So children listen to what we tell them. While this is true, children will learn very powerful messages from what we as parents *do*. We can tell them that soft drinks and chips are not good for them, but it will be a very weak message if we ourselves regularly consume junk food and soft drinks. While you might solace yourself that you have all of your adult teeth, you have stopped growing, that you're finally a 'grown-up' and *that's* why you can have cola while they drink milk, children don't see it that way. The whole 'It's not fair' game begins and children become drawn to those 'sometimes' foods and drinks like a magnet.

If you're serious about your family's diet, it is time to examine your own eating and drinking habits as well. Remember, *you* decide what food and drink comes into your house. If you don't want them to eat chocolate, don't bring it into the house in the first place. If you want them to choose healthy snacks, make sure there are plenty of these in the pantry and the fridge so that they can make good choices. People are more inclined to eat fruit that has been cut up than left whole. So leave small containers of cut-up fruit in the fridge. In short, make it easy for them to choose foods and drinks that will keep them healthy, happy and growing.

Mixed messages about food

Without realising it, we can send children other messages about food. One little girl came crying to Mum after grazing her knee. Mum cuddled her and encouraged her to go back and play. The little girl looked Mum in the eye and asked where her ice block was. Mum looked confused. The little girl explained that Mum always gave her an ice block when she cried. Mum blushed; she had no idea that this was a regular occurrence. The idea of distracting her child from the grazed knee was great, but the tool used to do the distracting needs some more thought. Similarly, parents may try to encourage their child to do a boring task, like tidying up their toys, with the reward of morning tea or lunch. Now the food may be very healthy, but the child learns that doing an unpleasant job can be paired with food. We see here that food is a mighty motivator. 'Forbidden foods' such as lollies or chocolate can become elevated in status if used as rewards for certain desirable behaviours. If we, as parents, can remember that food is fuel for our body and to treat it as such, we will help to reduce confusion and mixed food messages for developing little minds and habits.

Parents lie

Parents do one of the things they tell their children not to do; they lie. 'Just take a bite, Matthew.' Matthew takes a bite. 'See, that wasn't so bad. Now eat that entire cucumber boat.' One articulate child asked why she should take a bite in the first place. She explained that she knew the expectation was that she would have to eat the whole item regardless of whether she liked it or not, so why even try? Imagine being handed an awful assignment at work with the promise that if you completed it, it would be passed on to someone else next time. Imagine then how you would feel if your boss decided that you did the job well and you could do that awful job all the time. Would you feel like putting your hand up for more?

'Moving the goal posts' is another phrase that comes to mind. Imagine that you've been set a sales target of 70 per cent for the year with the carrot of a Christmas bonus for reaching your target. You reach the 70 per cent mark in October and the boss decides to change the annual target to 85 per cent. How would you feel? Children do not like it when you change your expectations midstream. Coach, when you are getting started on a new drill, take it one step at a time. Give older children information about what you expect of them at *this* meal. Today I want you to take a bite. They take a bite, and this is success all around. The game is over and both coach and player have won round one. The next night you can explain that, now, you want them to have three bites. When your child eats the three bites, again coach and player have won and the game is finished. Set the expectation at the beginning and then stick to it so that you both know when you've achieved your goal and you build trust.

Remember also that gradual changes are far easier to manage than big ones. Fussy eating habits have developed over a number of years with older children. They will not disappear overnight, in a week or even in a month. With persistence they will change, however, and certainly a snapshot of their diet today, and another snapshot in 12 months time, should show some fairly marked changes.

Parents make a fuss

Yes, you read that correctly, *we* make a fuss about food. If they eat a new food and enjoy it, there's a song and dance about 'See, aren't you glad you tried it!' maybe even with a little click of the heels thrown in. When they don't like a food or won't try it, there's a different scenario: 'Why won't you try it? You might just like it. Ohh I get so frustrated with you . . .' and silently the parent is foot stamping and mentally throwing their own mini tantrum because their child is not doing as they have asked. We need to relax about food, then the novelty of food being able to push Mum or Dad's buttons will disappear.

Eating to feel satisfied

A consistent comment from many adults is their recollection of being told to finish what was on their plate. For the children and grandchildren of parents who lived through the war, the message was particularly strong. In times of war there are food shortages. The patterns ingrained during those times of watching every cent, being careful with water consumption, and being careful with food purchased and eaten was critical to survival. Children were told to 'finish their plate' because their parents could not be certain of food supplies. In the decades following the war though, food was more plentiful. The demand to 'finish the plate' lived on to at least two more generations. While there are survival reasons to finish the plate during war times, the request to finish the plate in plentiful times leads to other complications.

Children often have little control over the amount of food that is served up to them. Pushing for them to finish every skerrick of food will result in full-on stand-offs if your child is already full. Eating more than they need to makes them feel uncomfortable. They learn to finish the plate to win Mum or Dad's approval rather than for its nutritional benefit. Children do not develop the important habit of listening to their own unique body for it to tell them when they are comfortably full or sated. Issues with increased weight occur when people eat more than they need to. When parents provide a range of healthy foods, it is reasonable to request a child try all of the different foods on the plate to increase their food variety. However, following this process, children should be allowed to determine how much they wish to eat that day. Parents will need to understand that their children's appetite may vary from week to week and will not be stable until they have stopped growing. By this stage they might just be moving out of home!

Food rewards

'If you eat all your broccoli you can have some jelly and ice-cream.'
At some stage we have all tried to bribe our children to eat their broccoli by offering them ice-cream as a reward. This 'may' work with your little one in the family; however, older fussy children are not so easily bribed. The bottom line is—don't bribe with treat foods. It is better to negotiate with the older child. Set them a clear non-food goal that they can aim for at the end of each week. You can give soft reminders to keep them on track, such as 'If you keep trying the new things I put on your plate, you can have a play-date with a friend, or we can go out to dinner to the restaurant of your choice.' This is far more positive than the alternative of fighting at the dinner table and forcing your child to eat. Telling your child that they will sit there until every morsel is eaten may work for the odd few children; however, most rebel and clamp their jaw shut even tighter. The key to an older child's heart is reward and recognition. Remember, it is all about them! Movies, plays in the park, play-dates or a sleep-over with friends are all great motivating rewards that don't cost a fortune or sacrifice other family activities. Putting the family holiday on the line not only sacrifices the

rest of the family but also gives the child in question way too much power. Be very careful what you bargain with, because you should always follow through!

HELPING CHILDREN TO UNDERSTAND *WHY* THEY HAVE TO EAT CERTAIN TYPES OF FOODS

At around three to four years of age children are full of wonder, asking questions about 'Why is the sky blue?' or 'Where does cream come from?'. If they have questions about 'why' they need to eat their fruit, vegetables, meat, cheese and other foods, it pays to be well-informed. Older children are beginning their journey into the age of reason. The first step in acceptance for many older children is an understanding of what the food is used for.

Chapter 3 gives information on what constitutes a good diet and that the variety of foods we eat is the essence to what will keep us healthy. While you, as an adult, understand why a good diet is important, it can be hard to explain this to children. Below you will find sections on food analogies. These sections give some ideas on how to explain the importance of a variety of foods in ways that children can understand.

Creative ways of explaining the importance of food variety

Many children spend their early years listening to stories. They have a fabulous imagination and a real sense of wonder with the world. We can now use our imagination and think creatively to help them better understand how food works. Sometimes you have to be quite creative in the way you sell a food. There are some general analogies and others that seem to be more gender-specific.

Earlier we talked about the stomach being a bit like a petrol tank. If you only put a little bit of petrol in the car, it will run out quickly and will slow down and eventually stop and need refuelling.

This kind of analogy can help children to understand the importance of breakfast for putting the first load of petrol into the tank, to get the car going. Regular pit stops happen every few hours as the tank runs low. We know that the tank is running low when the 'car' starts to go slower and break down (i.e. children get tired and cranky). For younger children, you can tie this information into their play. Run a small car along a play set and show them how the car needs to stop and needs more fuel. Then explain that the car is just like them, they also need to stop and refuel. Also remind children that just as we use sunscreen to protect the *outside* of our bodies, we use fruit and vegetables to protect the *inside* of our bodies.

Explaining to boys

Try telling a boy that eating eggs is going to help his nails grow and he is likely to turn and run in the opposite direction. Explaining that eggs are excellent for muscle growth, and will help him with his running and swimming, will be more successful when it comes to his enthusiasm for eating them. Young boys are often into fighter pilots and Star Wars characters. Explaining that fruit and vegetables are fighters that keep the bad bugs away can tap into familiar scenarios for them. Explaining that the fighter pilots can help them to stay healthy enough to play soccer or play with their mates on the weekend can do wonders.

Older boys may benefit from the following 'car engine' explanation. Engines run best on very pure, clean fuel. Put dirty fuel into an engine and the engine starts to malfunction. Our 'sometimes' foods and drinks, eaten in excess, can make the fuel 'dirty' and run less efficiently. A balance achieved with fruit, vegetables, legumes, protein, dairy and carbohydrates helps the tank to run efficiently and for children to grow well mentally and physically. Older boys are also interested in strength and muscles. Teenage boys triple their muscle mass during puberty. This helps to explain why they eat so much! Some parents of teenage boys have found that whilst their youngster was quite picky, a whole new world of food variety has been opened up—with the overwhelming urge to eat everything in sight—to their sons during puberty.

Explaining to girls

While young girls tend not to be amused by fighter pilots, they are often interested in fairies. The good fairies and bad fairies have magic wands, so where do they get their magic? They must eat lots of fruit and vegetables and other healthy foods! Girls are also more interested in their appearance than boys. Your 4-year-old daughter may wolf down yoghurt if she knows that her hair will grow long and shiny. Use the same approach to find out what is important for your 10-year-old daughter, and promote the foods she needs. Shiny hair, strong nails and clear skin may be motivation enough to help older girls to choose healthy foods.

General analogies and explanations

Food can be likened to fuel for a fire. We know that you need lots of different things to get a fire started and then to keep it going. Logs are a good source for long burning, while paper burns fast and disappears very quickly. Talk about a few foods and work out which foods are logs, which are paper, twigs and so forth. For example, logs might be things like meat, protein and dairy foods. Branches and kindling might be nuts, vegetables and fruit. Twigs might be crackers. Paper might be chips, chocolate, lollies, soft drink, etc.

Children from the age of six understand these concepts. As parents we can engage them to make good choices. Explain what is on their dinner plate or snack plate in terms of paper, branches, twigs and logs and encourage them to make choices for 'their fire'. Explaining that they will need some 'logs' so that they can concentrate at school, or swim fast, can give them a reason to eat the food other than to please their parents. As noted above, the concept of high and low GI foods could also be thought of in terms of fast burning and slow burning foods. Relating foods to a fire and what you use to build a fire provides a really concrete way for children to understand the concept.

How do you teach a child that iron found in protein is most effective when paired with vitamin C? Most children enjoy a piggyback ride. Children can be taught that fruit and vegetables give other foods (e.g. protein) a 'piggyback' to where those important foods need to go. The fruit and vegetables are 'helper' foods.

How do you teach a child the early fundamentals of cholesterol and plaque building up in blood vessels? One young fellow was fascinated with the blue lines on his arms—his veins. A discussion about blood and where it went and what it did followed. We talked about how blood flows through the blue lines because the blue lines are like little hoses. We talked about the garden hose and what happens when it gets blocked or damaged. We decided that clean hoses were really important. We talked about foods that could clog the hoses and worked out that these were 'sometimes' foods. Providing small reminders about keeping the hoses clean was all that was required when explaining that a doughnut was not a healthy choice for an afternoon snack.

THE OLDER CHILD'S GUIDE TO TRYING NEW FOODS

In Chapter 4 we looked at the steps to trying a new food. For younger children pairing the steps to trying a new food with a game work well. While some older children might also enjoy a game, you might only need to use the game for the first couple of times. An abridged version of steps to trying new foods for the older child is included in the following table.

Table 23: **Trying new foods—the older child**

Step	Activity	Reason
1	Touch the food. This might be using one finger to poke it gently and then progressing to picking it up and putting it back on the plate.	Touching the food gives you information about food texture. Fingertips are sensitive and provide some early indications of what food might feel like in the mouth.
2	Smell the food.	Aroma is one part of the two-part process of an appreciation of flavour. The way a food smells gives a very good indication of what it will taste like.
3	Touch the food to your lips (for younger children this is 'kiss the food').	The lips are very sensitive. Because of this sensitivity they work as the first gate as to whether to allow food to progress further into the mouth.
4	Touch your tongue to the food (for younger children this is 'lick the food').	The tongue, particularly the tongue tip, is super-sensitive. The tongue is the second gate to determining whether food will progress further.
5	Take one fingernail-sized piece of food and place it on the chewing surfaces of the molar teeth (choose left or right) and chew.	The teeth have pressure detectors, but are not as sensitive to texture as the lips and tongue. After chewing the texture of the food changes. Many children are happy to swallow the food because of the small size. If your child does not wish to

Step	Activity	Reason
		swallow the food, provide a napkin and show them how to politely remove it from their mouth. There is no spitting allowed!
6	Take a fingernail-sized piece of food and put it in the mouth, allowing the child's tongue to move it over to the tooth surfaces for chewing. Encourage your child to chew and swallow the food (two pieces on day two, three pieces on day three). By day four you can begin to place the new food, in the same small quantity, on the dinner or snack plate.	Having felt the texture from step 5, it is now time to re-engage the more sensitive part of the mouth, starting with the tongue. Keeping the pieces small makes them easy to chew. Small numbers of pieces makes the process achievable. Achievement builds confidence and success.
7	Take a bite of the food, chew and swallow.	This final step in the process re-engages the lips and tongue in the process of taking a bite of food. The whole process is complete with lips, tongue, chewing and swallowing now involved.

Remember to keep expectations in check. On day one you might get as far as having your child put their tongue onto the food. For the very fussy, just smelling the food might be an achievement. On a great day they might eat the one small morsel offered. The absolute pinnacle on day one is to have them chew and swallow one piece of the fingernail-sized piece of food. You can step it up to two bites the next day and so forth. While you might think this is like cutting the lawn with a pair of scissors, the approach works well using these very small but achievable goals. Aim to spend no longer than five minutes on this task. Following the activity, spending some time with your child, by playing a game or just talking about their day, is important. It doesn't have to be long, but it will mean the world to them. They have done something difficult. You can help them to feel more like repeating the process if you spend time with them afterwards, by showing them that *they* are important to you, not just getting them to eat a new food.

ESTABLISHING NEW HABITS

Deciding to change your child's diet is one of the biggest steps to developing the new habit of healthy eating. As noted many times, fussy eaters do not suddenly appear one day, they develop slowly over time. Children are also born with few innate food and flavour preferences.[2] These also develop over time and with repeated exposures. Developing new food habits takes months and it is important to have reasonable expectations. We have seen forlorn children who have eaten a sliver of apple for the first time in their lives being coddled, coerced or bullied into eating the rest of the apple on the way home in the car. To their horror the apple then appears in the lunchbox for days thereafter. These same well-meaning parents will phone a week or two later saying that the therapy didn't work, and that their child will not eat apple for them, only for the clinician. The 'take a bite and you own the carrot farm' concept is akin to asking someone to swim the English Channel when the most they have ever managed was a 25 metre dog paddle.

Clear and consistent communication is important with the older child. Have you noticed that people are inclined to become cranky when their appointment time has come and gone and there is no sign that they will be attended to any time soon? People are able to cope better if they are politely informed of how long they have to wait. For children, along with 'Are we there yet?', the other great phrase is 'How much do I have to eat?' Set an achievable goal at the beginning of the meal and then stick to your word. Your child will learn to trust you.

Habits are simply patterns of behaviour. They are performed so often that they become automatic and easy. Make it easy for yourself and your children by getting rid of things that will make it harder to establish a new habit. For example, ensure there are only healthy food choices in the pantry and the fridge. Turn the television off and eat dinner together at the table. Start with just one small change. For example, adding one new vegetable to the plate. Trying to change everything at once is akin to realising that you are travelling the wrong way down a freeway, stopping dead in the middle and doing a screaming u-turn. Your participants will be fearful! Change direction gradually and the participants will barely notice the change in scenery. As a general rule of thumb, it takes about 21 days to establish a new habit. To establish a new habit you first need to have identified the bad habits. Try writing the bad habits down so that it is easy to spot them. Establishing a new habit will take discipline and consistency on your part, even when you are tired and don't feel like it. And, finally, it will take patience and time.

Some people find it helpful to adopt the 'rule of three' when establishing a new habit: 'I am going to make a concerted effort to include carrot for three days.' Day one is good because you are full of enthusiasm. Day two may be harder, but you console yourself there is only one more day to go. Day three is generally easier to manage, as it is the finish line. Day four is a day of rest. If you stop now though, you are unlikely to be successful. Time to recommence on the next three days. Once you've managed the rule of three on two occasions, it is time to stretch it out to five days then take a one-day break. Following this, progress to seven days before a break. It doesn't all have to be the same food either. You might do carrots for the first three days and strawberries for the next three days. Once children understand the pattern, or the 'rules', they will become more tolerant participants.

NO ONE LIKES BEING TOLD WHAT TO DO

Even adults dislike being told what to do. You might meet a friend for coffee and relate a problem with your boss at work. Your friend sees this as an opportunity to show you how clever they are by solving your problem for you. Many people bristle when they feel someone else is telling them how to do something. It implies that they can't think for themselves. As children get older, similar situations arise. When they were younger, we did have to make their decisions for them. We dressed them, bathed them and fed them, and they happily cooperated. As they get older they are developing their own thinking skills and they want to exercise their decision-making abilities. The 'You will eat this because *I said so*' routine wears thin.

Following the 3-year-old age of 'why', you may have more success with your child if you engage them as a 'thinking' individual. Use the analogies provided above to give them information that helps them to make healthy choices for themselves. Once children have been provided with some information about different foods, ask them to 'teach' an adult what they've learned. This is a good way to work out what they have retained and helps to reinforce what they have learned.

MANAGING TAKEAWAYS AND SOFT DRINK

'Everything in good measure.' We've heard this statement about red wine and chocolate. And yes, there is a place for takeaway foods and soft drinks. We don't live the life of monastic monks and we would be lying if we said that we don't enjoy the occasional chocolate after dinner! If children are desperate for fish and chips or spring rolls, organise a date for it. It may be a regular occurrence like once a month, or as a special treat when they have been working hard at making good choices during the week. Healthy takeaway options include sushi, thin crusty wholegrain pizza, tomato-based pasta and Mexican dishes, to name a few. However, note also that children who are regular takeaway diners have been found to have more of an appetite for soft drink and high fat foods, and a correspondingly reduced consumption of fruits, vegetables and milk.[3] Keep takeaways and soft drinks for special occasions and emergency measures.

A GENTLE INTRODUCTION TO DINING AWAY FROM HOME— NEIGHBOURHOOD DINNERS

It has been said by many wise people that it takes a village to raise a child. With fragmentation of today's society, families do not always live close by. Building friendships with parents in your street or local neighbourhood can be beneficial on many levels. Both Kate and Julie have regular neighbourhood dinner engagements. The children thoroughly enjoy the chance to play at someone else's house and for parents it is a welcome and enjoyable social outing. You might have fortnightly or monthly get-togethers at alternate houses. You might have the host prepare the main meal for the evening while the guests bring a bottle of wine and some pre-dinner nibbles or fruit platter.

Neighbourhood dinners allow children an opportunity to try foods at other people's houses, in the company of other children. It is amazing how a 'pack mentality' can emerge. Watch the visiting children sneaking furtive glances at the inhabitants of the house to see how they put a spring roll wrapper together. Watch the children devour their mum's dinner. Visiting children are out of their usual comfort zone and are often encouraged to use their manners and to try something new. These opportunities allow children a stepping-stone to flying solo when they are invited to a friend's for a sleep-over. Mum or Dad is not there then to provide prompts on behaviour and manners around the dinner table. The lessons learned at neighbourhood dinners will stand them in good stead for a lifetime.

SCHOOL CAMPS AND SLEEP-OVERS

School camps can be anxiety-provoking for children because they do not know what to expect and what they can *imagine* can be fairly terrifying! There's sleeping away from home in a strange place, with strange sounds. There's hanging out with your classmates and teacher 24 hours a day. Then there's the food. Many a call has been put through to parents from the school campsite asking for help regarding their darling 7-year-old who has gone on a hunger strike. If you feel that your child will not cope, then maybe it is not the right time to send them off to battle. This could be something to work towards when getting them to try new things at home. The reward for trying ten new foods could be joining their friends for fun on the school camp.

For some children the thought of eating 'unknown' pizza, fish and chips or hamburgers can be overwhelming. It is important to help them understand that it is similar to food at home, possibly just prepared in a different way. Brief your child before they go off to camp or a friend's place for dinner or a sleep-over. Let them know that they will be required to eat with others and try something that they may be unfamiliar with. Children who have been taught how to try new foods will be in a far more comfortable position when away from home. They can be confident when trying new foods and make decisions for themselves on what food they will eat. Having been exposed to healthy choices at home, it is easier to make healthy choices away from home.

As children get older, some school camps have children cook for themselves. We have heard from one boys' school that the 'coolest boy' on camp was not the one who canoed the fastest, had the best ropes course time or told the best jokes. The 'camp legend' was the boy who could cook dinner! Parents, encourage boys to hang out in the kitchen. Start by just chatting with them about their day while you cook dinner. As time goes on, ask them to help out and accept whatever offers of help they proffer. There is something very rewarding about a 9-year-old who can cook a spaghetti dinner 95 per cent independently! You just don't know whether those skills will see them with the tag of 'coolest kid on camp' one day.

PATTERNS OF EATING FROM SCHOOL AGE TO 18 YEARS— MOTIVATION FOR CHANGING TO HEALTHY EATING HABITS

Research shows us that the number of different foods a child eats at around two to three years of age will likely predict the number of foods a child eats at eight years of age.[4] The literature also suggests that children aged two to six years of age may be harder to convince to try new foods. Enter the school system and children's relative aversions seem to slowly decrease. In fact, after 17 years of age, adolescents will be more inclined to spontaneously try different foods. There are also windows of opportunity between the ages of 8–12 years and 17–22 years. The terror teenage years of 13 to 16 yielded low results on the new food stakes. Researchers suggest that peer social groups, and a focus on height and weight, are likely to influence the shift in adolescents' tendencies to try new foods. Note, though, that the increases in the variety of foods sought is fairly modest and suggests that many food habits are well-ingrained by the time children are four years of age.[4]

In adolescence, boys tend to increase the variety and amount of meat products they consume. Decreased meat consumption in teenage girls has been noted by a number of researchers.[4] Children's vegetable repertoire at around two to three years of age was fairly predictive of the variety of vegetables they would eat through their teenage years. After about 17 years of age, adolescents seem to be more inclined to try different vegetables. The 'age of reasoning' may explain these findings, in that the benefits of vegetables and an increased awareness of weight, may influence food preferences in the latter teenage years. Similarly, patterns of dairy intake at around two to three years were strongly linked to dairy intake in the teenage years. Interestingly the 2–3-year-old's demand for bland starchy foods does not predict a later preference for starchy foods.

Recent Australian trends are worrying. A 2007 Australian National Children's Nutrition and Physical Activity Survey[3] found that intake of fruit and vegetables was higher in children aged four to eight years compared with teenagers (14–16 years). Sugar consumption increased with age. Australian State surveys indicate that one in six children have inadequate levels of vitamin C and half of all children surveyed had inadequate vegetable consumption, shown by inadequate potassium levels. Vitamin C is important as it maximises the benefits of iron in the diet. Potassium is essential to keep muscles, nerve cells, the heart and the kidneys functioning well. Regular consumption of potassium-rich food helps to keep your heart in good working order as you age. Girls aged ten to 15 years had inadequate iron levels. Iron is an essential mineral and important for energy and brain development due to its role in moving oxygen around the body. Calcium intake was insufficient in half of 10–15-year-olds, with the intake for girls particularly problematic. Calcium is the main mineral present in both bones and teeth. Children aged nine to 18 years need more calcium than toddlers and adults in order to fuel bone growth during growth spurts throughout puberty. The study also showed that soft drink consumption increased as children grew older.

Whilst many younger children regularly eat breakfast, this tendency drops off as children reach their middle teenage years. Girls seem to skip breakfast more often than boys. Also, about 30 per cent of teenagers did not eat lunch daily. Dinner was the meal most likely to be eaten by teenagers. Our busy lifestyles are also beginning to show their effects. For most children and teenagers, a dinner where all of the family was present happened on four nights of the week. Fruit and vegetable intake is best in families that eat together. Eating dinner in front of the TV showed an increase in convenience foods and a drop in fruit and vegetable intake.[3,5,6] Pleasantly though, fewer than 20 per cent of children were having takeaway food weekly. Frequency of takeaway meals tended to increase in families with a low socioeconomic status.

DISORDERED EATING—ANOREXIA AND OBESITY

The 2007 Australian National Children's Nutrition and Physical Activity Survey[3] found that 72 per cent of children surveyed were a healthy weight, 17 per cent of boys and girls were classified as overweight, 6 per cent were obese, and 5 per cent were underweight. The eating disorders of anorexia nervosa and obesity fall at either end of the spectrum. On one hand you have parents beside themselves as they watch their child literally wasting away, while the other hand shows a child whose excessive food intake places them at risk of diabetes and heart disease. These conditions are serious. Assistance from medical and nutritional professionals is important. Often psychological counselling is also recommended.

Parents can assist children in a number of ways. Ensure that there are opportunities for good food choices at home. It is easier to choose fruit, vegetables, yoghurt or nuts as a snack if there are no chips, lollies, chocolates or biscuits to tempt them otherwise. As much as possible, have meals together as a family. It is easier to spot a change in eating habits if there is a familiar routine. Family meals also provide a chance to talk about what else is going on in children's lives. If children are finding social aspects difficult, they may eat to 'feel better'. An ability to draw this to their attention and provide alternatives may help prevent a bad habit from taking hold. As noted previously, avoid asking children to 'finish their plate'. Children may eat all on their plate to please you, or to win your love and approval. Instead, encourage children to listen to their body cues of hunger and feeling 'comfortably full'. These are important skills to have and help foster confidence in their decision-making and the reality of consequences. 'If I choose not to eat dinner,

I am likely to be hungry later on and I know there is nothing more till breakfast.' This scenario probably only need play out once for children to learn a valuable ancient survival message. Many parents are too fearful to let a child skip a dinner meal even once. This fear seems irrational when we consider that during illness children's food intake diminishes considerably.

Obesity

Obesity is fast becoming a serious problem in Australia. Standardised height and weight charts are typically derived from sampling a large number of children. Researchers updating growth charts have recently been faced with a new dilemma. How do you plot a population's average height and weight without making obesity seem 'normal'? Children who are obese are more at risk of going on to be obese adults. Children with two obese parents are more likely to become obese than children of two thin parents.

Researchers are still trying to determine the exact links between genetics and influence of the environment in which children grow up as to the causes of obesity. Certainly children who are exposed to many high-fat and energy-dense foods, with few opportunities to try fruits and vegetables, will, by law of nature, develop a tendency towards the foods most on offer and most frequently sampled. If we imagine a car with a 40 litre fuel tank that travels a short distance only once a day, the fuel tank will not need regular topping up. A car's fuel tank will overflow and cause a mess, making it obvious to the owner that no more fuel is required. The same is not true of humans, however; humans do not begin to vomit when their 'fuel tank is full'. The body has to do something with the excess and so stores it for times of famine. In the prosperous age in which we live, the need for fat stores is low.

Overweight and obese children have been found to have different eating patterns to children in the healthy weight range. Specifically, children in the healthy weight range regularly eat three meals a day. Children who were obese had sporadic meal habits.[6] It is possible that overweight children deny themselves meals in order to reduce their weight, or may snack regularly on inappropriate foods, such that they are not hungry at regular mealtimes. Skipping breakfast is also associated with obesity.[6] Eating a healthy breakfast has been shown to provide increased concentration at school, better cognitive function, social interaction, nutrient balance and energy levels. Obesity is more often found in teenagers who do not eat a regular dinner meal and those from a low socioeconomic background. In contrast, children who eat dinner regularly with their family have been shown to have lower levels of obesity. Interestingly, research has also found that children who eat with their family tend to have lower levels of soft drink consumption.

Apart from the type and amount of food consumed, there is another important factor. We will burn more fuel (food) when we move and exercise more. This is like our little car having a regular 100 km drive. The need for fuel increases. While making healthy choices about the type of foods eaten and the amount of food eaten is important, another vital factor is exercise. Burn the fuel that is taken in and also mobilise the stored fuel. Exercise can be very difficult for people who are overweight as their bones are supporting masses more than they were designed to. These people tire easily and may become disheartened with the task at hand. People do not go to bed thin one night and wake up the next morning overweight or obese. It happens very slowly over time. Removing the unwanted weight will also happen slowly and over time with discipline and determination. Assistance from an accredited practising dietitian, an exercise trainer or gym are necessary support networks for successful weight reduction and establishing healthy habits. Earlier in this chapter we discussed information about recommendations for physical exercise for children.

Anorexia

Children who are underweight may be more prone to illness and more easily fatigued. They may have lower levels of concentration and may be more irritable. Children as young as eight years of age are being hospitalised and treated for malnutrition. An extreme end of this spectrum is anorexia nervosa. Anorexia sits at the other end of a parent's nightmare. This is a serious medical condition that goes well beyond food. Body image is distorted to the point where people with this disorder do not see themselves as underweight or even skeletal in appearance. Adolescents are at highest risk of developing this disorder.

The person with anorexia fears getting fat. Their parents fear for their nutrition and long-term health. It is sobering to note that death related to anorexia occurs at a rate 12 times higher than the standard mortality rate.[7] Even following recovery there are long-term issues relating to osteoporosis.[8] Most of our bone mass is acquired by our second decade of life. In females, in particular, there is limited bone-mass acquisition from two years after they start menstruation. As such, the timing of anorexia can rob girls of critical bone density. Poor bone density means that bones are more likely to fracture. As noted above, calcium intake is critical for assisting with bone development. Girls need to be encouraged to increase their intake of calcium-rich foods to keep their bones strong in later life.

Anorexia is a complicated disorder and often involves the dedicated support of a team. The team provides medical management for re-feeding, nutritional support for nutritional recovery, and psychological support for recovery relating to anxiety. Those with anorexia also benefit from strategies to reintegrate with society while rebuilding their own perceptions of themselves. The re-feeding process is in itself tricky. Few understand that the initial weight gains are fluid. Without continued nutritional support, this initial weight gain does not convert over to lean body mass. People with anorexia can initially gain several kilograms whilst hospitalised, but lose all weight gain within a few days if they don't continue to take sufficient kilojoules.[7] Researchers advise that sustained and controlled nutritional support over six to 12 weeks is critical to the recovery of lean body mass, also known as muscle mass.

Tips for shopping, cooking, lunchboxes and others

It's fascinating how meals 'work'. You spend an hour in the kitchen to prepare a meal, ten minutes to eat it and then another half hour to clean up the kitchen again. Of course, just to keep things interesting there's always the scenario of preparing that same meal and having small people whinge and moan. There's also the joy of throwing their uneaten food in the bin. In an age where we are determined to reduce our carbon footprint and 'go green', less wastage is best for the environment as well as the cranky cook! This chapter includes some straightforward ways to reduce dinner food wastage.

Then there are the lunches. For most mums, the children's excitement about the holidays is matched closely by their own excitement about not having to fill lunchboxes every day! Kate and Julie are both working mums. Both have primary-school aged children, but have also had experience with childcare, nannies, kindergartens, preschools and schools. This chapter includes practical tips, tried and true, for the busy household; that is, every house that contains children!

PLANNING FOR THE WORKING FAMILY

Life has changed considerably over the past 40 years. It is very common to find either both parents working or single parent families. Mealtimes can be the straw that breaks the camel's back after a long day at work before beginning the evening shift on the home front. Organisation is the name of the game. A few lists and plans won't go astray if all members or carers in the family are working. Whether you are full-time, part-time or casual there will be a few days a week where you will feel like the day is an army manoeuvre. Planning your weekly meals is essential and making sure two or three of them can be used as leftovers some time during the same week takes the pressure off having to cook up a storm every night. Tip number one is to make sure you check you have everything for dinner before you leave for work in the morning. If you are strapped for time, pack kids' lunchboxes the night before or make a week's worth of lunches and freeze them. Do any baking on the weekend, and include the kids in the process. Write a shopping list using evening meal plans and lunchbox grids to plan your shopping. This will allow you to grocery shop once per week for everything with only small top-ups as needed.

HAPPINESS IS A ROUTINE

Planning meals is a good way of setting routines and, yes, children thrive on routines. Some children feel safe in the fact that Monday night is 'burrito night' and Friday is 'homemade pizza night'. They look forward to their favourites and are more comfortable knowing when the 'new meals to try' are coming. The power of choice is also important. If you like a bit more variety, ask each family member to nominate a favourite meal. To start with it may look like a takeaway menu, but with some clever negotiations you can build a healthy weekly menu. The resounding favourite of all three Cichero children is spinach cannelloni. Some weeks there are feverish negotiations between the younger members of the household as to whether there will be Indian or Mexican on the menu that week.

You could place the weekly food planner on the fridge with a few pictures for junior members of the household. A piece of paper with the menu plan for the week ahead can just be written up and stuck to the fridge for the literate members of the household. This small step allows children to work up to the meals, knowing there are no 'surprise attacks' of unfamiliar foods coming in when they least expect it. It also allows children to check ahead of time and answer the grating question of 'What's for dinner tonight Mum?'

You may be sitting back right about now thinking 'What fairyland are these parents living in?!' However, if meals are being rejected night after night, give it a try; your children may pleasantly surprise you. All of these tricks of the trade, including menu plans (see below) and scrapbooks, are just constantly reminding them of what foods exist. When they see meals on their plates that are familiar, they are more inclined to eat them. As your child gets older they can start picking a meal and be involved in the planning, preparation and cooking of the meal. This gives children ownership, and again they will be more likely to sample something of their own making.

MENU PLANNING HELPS WITH BUDGETS, TIME MANAGEMENT AND FOOD CHOICES

Planning weekly meals is a great way to budget. Some people shop in a state of semi-stupor barely aware of the items being placed in the trolley. Night after night, they then struggle with the dilemma of what to cook for dinner from what is in the fridge or pantry. This process possibly accounts for the prolific rise of cookbooks requiring fewer ingredients than the fingers on one hand. Write a shopping list and never be caught at 6.30 p.m. looking at hungry faces with no idea what to feed them. Parents find they fall into the trap of grabbing fish and chips or takeaway pizza, and these then become the familiar meals. Takeaway foods should be 'occasional' foods due to their high fat, high salt and low-fibre contents.

If you shop once a week, take the time to work out in advance what you are going to have for dinner each night. By doing this, you can purchase exactly what you need for the week ahead. You can also use this planning time to work out which vegies will go with each meal and also which fruits to get. Weekly shopping means good freezer and refrigerator space. Whether you shop once a week, once a fortnight or every three days, the process of menu planning can still be applied.

We hear many parents tell us that their children will only eat 'fish and chips' or 'biscuits and cola'. This may be hard to hear, but as parents *you* are in charge of the shopping list and what items are brought into your home. There are no kitchen fairies to magic up your child's dream foods. Food is fuel for the body. Put the wrong fuel or dirty fuel in and you will see some little engines that run poorly and backfire. In children we recognise this as difficult behaviour. Be strong, and after the initial kitchen cupboard door slamming and wailing on the floor, children will fall into step and slowly but surely the range and variety of foods they eat will grow. We have to be very careful with the fuel (food) we put into our bodies and those of the precious little people in our care.

Parental models are also important. Children will watch what you *do* and copy this rather than listen to what you *say*. It is difficult to explain to a child that it's okay for Dad to have a soft drink every night for dinner and to start the day with a chocolate bar, but not okay for them to do it. So, rule number one is to only purchase the things you would like your child to eat. For families with fully-fledged 'fussy eaters', meet this burden for a month before introducing the odd treat. Remind yourself and your child of what 'everyday' foods are and what 'sometimes' foods are, so that you are not tempted to fall back into bad habits.

GROCERY SHOPPING

Our world is full of stimuli. Wherever we go there are things to tantalise our tastebuds and stimulate our appetites. Bookshops and supermarket shelves display cookbooks, meal guides and magazines full of recipes helping us to plan, buy and cook our meals. They even say that recipe books are the 'modern woman's pornography'. However we look at it, visuals are important when planning our meals. Visuals are especially important when it comes to feeding children.

When children are faced with something they don't know, or have never seen, the answer will probably be 'no'. Young ones don't have the experience that adults do, so given a choice they will probably demand something that is familiar to them, like spaghetti or fish and chips, rather than stick their neck out and try something new. It doesn't matter if you are the queen of the up-sellers you will still probably get a resounding 'no'.

An easy way to breed familiarity is to show children meals in pictures. When planning the weekly meals (this can breakfast, lunch, dinner, snacks and lunchbox fillers), sit down with your children and give them a cookbook, recipe book or food style magazine to look at and pick something that they would like to try. Kids love the fact that you can make something that looks the same as the book. This also builds trust that it has arrived as expected. It is similar to our experiences in restaurants as an adult. Imagine picking a dish, having a pretty good idea of how it will look and taste, only to be disappointed when it arrives at the table, completely the opposite to what you expected. Children's reactions are no different. In many foreign countries there are pictures accompanying menus in restaurants to help us make meal decisions. So think of children as kind of like little foreign visitors dining in our restaurants.

Grocery planning

For the younger members of the household, make meal planning fun by collecting some supermarket brochures and food style magazines and have your children cut out various foods or meals. You can make a food-style bingo game, or they can paste their cut-out foods into a scrapbook with a theme. Themed pages such as foods starting with 'C' or red-coloured foods can then be taken to the supermarket and played like a treasure hunt. Smaller children will not have the words to tell you that they want the chicken risotto with the mushrooms and carrot. If you're feeling very pumped, why not take a digital photo of your child happily eating some of your family's regular meals and use them like a photo menu so that they can also contribute to the weekly menu planning. Another easy way of enticing children to try some new foods or complete meals is to cut out pictures of the foods and have them laminated so they double as placemats. You can tick off with a permanent pen or stamp with a star when each food has been attempted. Children can then proudly show off all of their little accomplishments to Grandma and Grandpa, for example.

Take a trolley and begin

Grocery shopping is painful at the best of times, and even more so when you have children trailing along behind. Bored children look for ways to entertain themselves. Fighting with siblings, rearranging products on shelves, and nagging for sweets and treats tick all the boxes for 'good entertainment' from a child's perspective. We teach children how to tie their laces and to get dressed, so why not teach them some life skills like how to grocery shop? The fruit and vegie department is a great place to start. For 2–3-year-olds, why not practise counting 'robust' vegetables (e.g. potatoes or carrots) as they go into the plastic bag. Robust vegetables work well while their handling skills improve! Teach them how to spot a good head of lettuce. Kids aged three and four can be taught to pick up fruit and smell it as they put it in the bag. Talk about the texture of the fruit and also the smell to give them some words to describe the aromas and what they are seeing and feeling. Talk about the different fruits that are available in summer versus winter. During summer teach children how to pick up and feel whether a peach is ripe and to smell it to see whether it has a sweet peachy aroma. Often the fruit that smells terrific tastes terrific. This is also an opportunity for children to touch and smell fresh food knowing that they will not be eating it right at that moment. These occasions will also have benefits in the future. They will ensure that when part-time jobs are on offer for teenagers that at least your child won't fall into the 20 per cent of checkout assistants that need to ask their customer to play 'identify the fruits and vegies' for them.

Older children can be given a small shopping list. Use items that are stored together (e.g. fruit and vegies) and give them their own basket to collect 'their' shopping list. You have taught them how to pick good fruit and vegetables, and taught them how to count, why not let them be in charge of that part of the shopping? You may still have to provide quality control from time to time to ensure that your standards are upheld, but that is a small price to pay for a child's growing independence and valuable life skills. More than one child; let them take turns to fill the basket and hand over to a sibling to load the contents into the trolley. Pass the empty basket to the next sibling and begin again. For variety why not try an early morning market where the food is the freshest you will find?

Avoid using sweets and treats as rewards for good behaviour whilst grocery shopping. We are delving back into the world of performing seals with that kind of caper! If the time is right for morning or afternoon tea, why not find a fruit smoothie, sushi or popcorn to refuel their tanks.

Once the grocery shopping is finished and all of those bags are sitting on your kitchen floor, children can again be part of the process of packing things away. To start with put them in charge of 'robust' items like tins, pasta and washing powder so that eggs are not splattered all over the floor. We have been known to practise rugby passing skills as items are passed from the bag to one child and then another before being passed to Mum or Dad to put them into the pantry. Fun for all the family! It sounds clichéd, but the task is over more quickly because many hands really do make light work.

COOKING

Have you noticed how the modern kitchen has become the central hub of the household? Gone are the days where Mum was busily preparing meals in the little room at the back of the house, usually adjacent to the laundry. Now the kitchen is large and where all the action takes place. The kitchen bench is large enough for adults to chat around, homework to be done on, and little children to sit at and learn to cook. It's time to get kids back into the kitchen. Children love to build and create things. Helping Mum or Dad from an early age is a wonderful time to bond and helps children to see how food is made. They see items of food in their individual whole forms before they are used as an ingredient in the meal. Better still, you can grow a few vegetables or salad items in the backyard. It is no myth that you have a greater chance of getting your children to try their homegrown items, especially if they are named after them: 'Look at Rosie's sugar snaps. Wow, they're so delicious!'

In 2002 a study was done which found that children recognised only a rudimentary number of fruits and vegetables. The fruits most readily recognised by children were apple, banana and grapes, but rarely rockmelon. Of the vegies, the carrots and tomatoes were the best recognised, but one in three children did not know what celery looked like[1]. We need to keep reinforcing the rule of two serves of fruit and five serves of vegetables per day. We recognise that some children have only two to three fruits and two to three vegetable or salad items that they are comfortable with. This can still be adequate. In time they will try others but always praise them for the ones they are eating.

Life skills, reading and maths—Benefits to children being involved in cooking

Even the youngest child can be involved in the cooking process. A toddler can be sat safely on a bench to watch as you weave your magic in the kitchen preparing the evening meal. Talking to them about what you are doing gives them new words to learn. Watching you peel or grate or cut shows them the special ways that foods can change shape. Little people can be involved by washing fruit or vegetables. If the child is about three years of age, you could let them try cutting a banana with a blunt plastic knife. Kinder and preschool children can learn to use the grater. To start with they may only be able to manage grating a small amount of the vegetable. They are using their hand muscles in a very different way to the way they've used them before. It will take practice to get better at grating and having the arm and hand strength to manage the job. Like everything in life though, it only gets better with opportunities to practise. Primary school kids can learn to use the peeler and with excellent supervision can be taught to safely use and respect a knife. Commonsense must prevail with use of blunt knives in soft foods before sharper knives and hard-textured foods are introduced.

The kitchen is a fabulous place to learn about maths and also reading. Showing children recipe books and getting them to find the ingredients can be like a pantry treasure hunt. Show them the word 'flour' on the page and then the word 'flour' on the packet. This early word matching and visual recognition of words will stand them in good stead as they learn to read at school. Cooking helps with maths. For little children, counting the biscuits on a baking tray or pikelets as they cook in a pan is a helpful introduction to counting; a cornerstone of mathematics. Counting two cups of flour or showing them that half a cup is different to a whole cup are concrete concepts that will help them in later years at school. Fractions can be discussed over an apple pie, a quiche or a pizza.

Promoting meal 'ownership' and encouraging involvement in cooking

Children involved in the preparation of a meal will take ownership and are particularly excited to present their triumph when the family sits down for dinner. If everyone makes a fuss over how nice the meal is, any reluctance to try from the young chef will soon disappear. Designate a cooking day per child to contribute their ideas and skills to help involve them in the cooking process. For example, children love to crack eggs (messy but fun), work the button on the food processor, or shell the peas. You can even buy children's aprons and miniature utensils for the budding Jamie Oliver in your household.

It is never too late to get your children into the kitchen as these skills are needed right through to adulthood. Remember the flatmate who survived on 'canned pies' and 'cup of noodles'? He's probably a frequent flyer at the local takeaway store. It pays to help children learn to be involved in meal preparation. We recognise, though, that it can be tricky to work out how to get started.

Everyone has their own way of helping. This is not to say that people always offer the kind of help you necessarily want at that particular moment in time. For example, when babies are newborn, one friend might make a dinner or a family member might do all the washing and ironing. This is all 'great help', unless what you really want is for someone to hold the baby while you escape for 15 minutes to hang the washing on the line by yourself! So how does this relate to children in the kitchen? When children ask 'Can I help?', embrace it! Accept every piece of 'help' offered if you want to continue enticing your child into the kitchen as they grow older. The benefits of a teenager who can take a turn at cooking dinner is a gift worth working for.

If your child offers to peel the cucumber, let them go for it. If they don't want to peel the carrot and potato, that's okay, just remember to say 'thanks for peeling the cucumber' and they will be more likely to come back and help again next time. When you graciously accept all offers, and also that it takes practice to get fast and really good at most kitchen jobs, children will happily wander through the kitchen, picking bits and pieces to help out with. This ad hoc approach does work. Milestones such as successful toilet training and children being able to put on their own seatbelts are followed closely by pre-teens who are budding cooks. It is a Kodak moment when your 9–10-year-old can cut her own fruit, make a spaghetti sauce with minimal instruction, and read a recipe book to produce a mean chocolate cake, only requiring help from a grown-up to get the cake into and out of the hot oven.

Freezer surprise

Dinners pose one of the biggest threats to household equilibrium. Parents, tired after a day at work, may feel like preparing dinner about as much as they would like to nail their hand to the floor. Some very organised people cook up a storm on the weekend and prepare meals that can be defrosted and reheated after work. Some people pay their nannies to cook a meal and have it ready waiting for them. Then there is 'freezer surprise'!

It is very difficult to predict exactly how much each person will eat for dinner each night and a plate of leftovers is common in most houses, excluding those with teenage boys! Preparing a little more and freezing a single serve is very do-able. Supermarkets now stock the plastic containers that we are so used to seeing at takeaway restaurants. These containers stack very well in the freezer. Over the course of a week or so, you gradually build up a supply of single-serve dinners. Freezer surprise means that each person can choose their own special dinner and arm wrestle or practise their debating skills for the favourites. Single serves are quick to heat in the microwave. You cooked them so you know that they are healthy, and it is easy to throw a salad together to go with these meals if required.

SCHOOL LUNCHES

Parents worry a great deal about children's lunchboxes. They worry about (a) how much food is in it, (b) whether their child will eat what is in it, (c) what the teacher will think of what they have put in the lunchbox, and (d) whether the lunchbox will come home from school, or disappear into the never-never of 'lost and found'. For most parents preparing school lunches is one of the most-hated chores of the 12 or so schooling years. Did you know that in an average year we make around 190 school lunches *per child* per year? No wonder we run out of ideas. The one thing that makes the hellish job so unrewarding is when the box comes home untouched and a tad smelly or there is evidence of 'wrappers' that were not there in the morning—the swapped lunch! Lunchbox food is different to food prepared and eaten at home. The food contained within needs to be robust enough to cope with being tossed around a school bag. Blackened bananas will turn off even very good eaters. In the Australian climate, lunchbox food also needs to be able to cope with heat. Although chicken, lettuce and cheese is a healthy choice, the sandwich should not look like it is incubating a new species of bacteria by lunchtime. Lunchbox food can be difficult.

A word of warning: Do not *ever* use the lunchbox to try out a new food for the first time! Your child will view the foreign item with all the appeal of a hand grenade and it will inevitably boomerang straight back to you. Lunchbox foods should be foods that the child has seen, touched, smelled, tasted and taken a few bites of before. Once they have done this in the safety of your home and with your cheering support, it is time to introduce the 'food challenge' to the lunchbox. The instructions are as follows: 'You remember rockmelon? It's orange and sweet and juicy. We had some yesterday afternoon. Today you have a food challenge. There is one piece of rockmelon in this container for you to eat at school. It will be so easy for you because you've done it before.' One piece is very achievable. The next day step it up to two pieces. By the time you hit five pieces they may even have stopped counting. Note: Keep the pieces about the size of your thumbnail. Children are not fooled by a 'piece' so big that it looks like it should have its own postcode.

What's in a healthy lunchbox?

Chapter 3, 'What is a good diet?' is a great place to start for healthy lunchbox fillers. The key to a good, healthy lunchbox is to provide slow release or low glycaemic index (GI) carbohydrate foods, such as multigrain bread or crackers and unpeeled fruits such as apples, grapes and strawberries. This will give children sustained energy and concentration throughout the day. A calcium-rich dairy food will sustain their appetite and provide important calcium for teeth and bones. Protein-rich meats, chicken, fish, eggs and legumes will provide valuable iron for transporting oxygen and zinc for the immune system.

There are many ready-made items available as 'healthy' lunchbox fillers; however, the reality is that many are high in fat and salt, or contain no real fruit or staying power. Many teachers report a room full of crazed little strangers once their class returns from lunch. This might just be due to the excessive intake of foods high in sugar and colours, or refined foods with no sustaining power. A 99 per cent fat-free fruit strap may appear to be a healthy lunchbox filler, but all it provides is enough fast-release sugar for a jet engine and the sticking power of superglue. This is not a great recipe for someone about to sit in a classroom for an hour and will also put a hole in your pocket with dental bills.

The lunchbox should contain:

- Water
- Fresh fruit/dried fruit
- Vegetable/salads such as carrot, celery, tomato
- Calcium-rich dairy foods such as milk, yoghurt, cheese

Wholegrain or wholemeal bread or crackers

Iron-rich proteins such as meat, fish, chicken, legumes, hommus and egg.

Healthy lunchbox snacks

You cannot go past a piece of fresh fruit. Fresh fruit is high in fibre, low in fat and salt, and provides slow-release carbohydrates for sustained energy. It is perfect for children and adults alike. Other healthy snacks for kids include dried fruit, yoghurt, low-fat cheese and crackers, wholemeal fruit scones or scrolls, popcorn and vegetable sticks with avocado dip or hommus.

Handling lunchbox boomerangs

Encourage children to bring all uneaten food home. If one particular food keeps reappearing, it allows us to ask for some feedback. 'I notice that the orange has been coming home the last two days? Did you want to tell me something about that?' Now sometimes the answer is that the child's just been too busy playing, while at other times they will tell you that they want to try something different. It works well to ask your child to nominate a healthy alternative to replace the rejected food. By working cooperatively, packing a lunchbox is less like a game of Mastermind and becomes more about straightforward communication.

Lunchbox packaging

For durability, investing in some good hard plastic containers helps to protect the food and also helps the environment by reducing packaging. Common themes for keeping lunchboxes cool include using small ice bricks and freezing drinks that defrost as the day goes on. Interestingly, many lunch foods can be prepared and frozen ahead of time. Pop the frozen morsels into lunchboxes at breakfast time and they will be defrosted and cool by first break. It is possible to spend only 45 minutes to make 18 lunches to freeze for the week ahead (we know because we've timed it as part of our own weekly routines). Anything from Vegemite, to cheese, to ham and chutney and even toasted cheese sandwiches can be made up and frozen for the week ahead. Use zip-lock bags and a marker pen to label people's lunches. Daily, fruit can be cut and frozen in small containers, even if only for a couple of hours before it goes into the lunchbox. Homemade 'treats' such as pikelets, fruit muffins, pieces of banana cake or scones can be stored in the freezer. Making lunches is easier to cope with on bleary-eyed mornings when the hardest task is reading the scrawl on the zip-lock bag to put the lunches into the right boxes.

A number of small boxes within the big lunchbox provides your child with some choices. If they are hitting a growth spurt, they may devour the lot and ask you why you didn't pack more. If they are cruising, they may eat most of what you've packed but not all of it. Providing just two large items can make lunchtime decisions daunting for a child. If they start to eat the enormous red apple but don't get it finished, it will be brown by the next break and unlikely to be eaten.

School breaks—The brain break

Many schools are leading the charge with fitness and healthy food choices. Some schools have introduced a 'brain break'/'fruit break'/'munch and crunch' break at about 10 a.m. in recognition that some children eat a very early breakfast meal. The first school break at around 11 a.m. is actually closer to lunch for a child's body clock than the later 1.30 p.m. break. So a healthy snack at about 10 a.m. can do wonders for children's concentration. There is also another benefit. Children have the opportunity to see their peers eating healthy 'everyday' foods. Like it or not, children are heavily influenced by the behaviour of those around them. This very sensible move by the education sector encourages strong, positive messages about healthy foods. Foods allowed during these special snack times generally include fruit (fresh, dried or tinned), vegetables and cheese. Be brave and think outside the box. It does not have to be just fruit. Some children love cucumber boats or a small container of cherry tomatoes.

'Fussy eaters' should be encouraged to take a bite. Teachers may benefit from reading some of the tips in Chapter 4 to see how they can encourage children to try new foods. Timid fruit eaters are often happier to start with dry fruits: Think sultanas or apricots that have been halved or quartered. It takes a fair bit of chewing strength to chew a dried apricot. After this, the 'very fussy' are often able to take on peeled apple as a first foray into the field of fresh fruit. Orange and, if in season, mandarin form the next part of the fruit dance before moving on to other fruits. Each child is different, however, so use tips from Chapter 4 to work out what might suit your child's needs best.

Kindergarten and preschool

This is the beginning of a structured peer influence on our children. They learn to move as a group from inside time to outside time and to sit on a mat. They learn about rules such as 'walking legs inside and running legs outside', and 'no hat—no play'. Children learn to eat at little tables and chairs and they get to peek inside their neighbour's lunchbox. Some kindies and preschools encourage families to bring a piece of fruit to contribute to a group fruit platter for morning tea. Often, small groups of children will be involved in washing, cutting or serving the fruit to their playmates. This approach is akin to what might happen at home in the kitchen and should be encouraged. Children may need some help learning how to try new foods. Patience, achievable goals and lots of encouragement are a must (see tips in Chapter 4).

Parents can follow the tips provided above for what to pack into the lunchboxes. Do be aware that little fingers are still learning how to open lids and handle containers. Imagine yourself trying to open up a tin of tomatoes with boxing gloves on! Giving children some practice at home will help them to become more confident and independent at kindy or preschool mealtimes.

Attention please preschool and kindy teachers! Research shows that if you are exuberant and excited about the food in the child's lunchbox, the child will be more likely to get it out and give it a go.[2] They will also be watching you to see what you are eating. Yes, expressing your own enjoyment of your fruit or salad *does* help young children to be brave enough to try these foods for themselves. If you are aware that some of your little charges are 'fussy eaters', separate them and sit each fussy eater at a table of 'good' eaters. The positive peer pressure has also been shown to help fussy eaters.[2] Sitting a group of fussy eaters together will only encourage fussy eating habits.

To the best of our knowledge 'fruit and vegetable breaks' are a school initiative that may not have filtered into kindergarten and preschool. Remember that these little people have little tanks. If children have had breakfast at 7 a.m., by the first break at 11 a.m. you will probably find yourself surrounded by irritable and irrational little people. It is amazing how putting food into their little systems at regular intervals will even out the crankies. In the meantime, parents please encourage your child to eat their sandwich or have their yoghurt at the first break so that they have enough energy to get through till the next break.

Nannies and other carers

Families with three or more children may have found it cheaper to have a nanny come to them rather than use childcare services. Nannies become important role models for your children. It is important that the nanny knows what types of food you want your children to eat and what times to serve the food. Any mealtime rules need to be clearly communicated. Different to the odd visit by aunts and uncles, these people cannot be Good Cop to your Bad Cop. This is a recipe for disaster. United we stand, divided we fall and the children dance all over us. Where grandparents are involved in your child's routine weekly care in the same way that a nanny or childcare centre might be, it is worth discussing your 'food' expectations. Children respond to different environments, so perhaps treats happen at Grandma and Grandpa's house, while regular meals and snacks are always on offer in the child's home. From a safety perspective, grandparents and other carers may also need a refresher on foods that pose a choking risk.

Childcare centres

Childcare centres run by very strict accreditation guidelines, including ratios for number of carers per child and the types of food offered. Dietitians and nutritionists are often involved in providing the guide-lines for foods served in childcare settings and after-school care settings. It is reasonable to ask to see what types of food are offered to children before deciding on your chosen centre. Some centres have been known to have very gourmet offerings. It may be worthwhile checking to see whether accommodation is made for children with a blander palate. Some centres have children bring packed lunchboxes. Although working parents are tired at the end of the day, children in long-day care will also be exhausted at the end of their busy day. Toddlers will hopefully be having a meal at around 5 p.m. or 5.30 p.m. at their childcare centre, so they may only be interested in a light snack (e.g. yoghurt) before bath and bed.

Lunchbox grids—Making life easier for the busy household

'I'm 1000 kilometres away from home, preparing to give two days worth of lectures and hoping that my lunchbox grid works for my husband as well as it works for me. 6.15 a.m. the following day this text message arrives: *U r a goddess - lunches r so easy! Just fruit and BAM! All done! Breakfast ready, reading headlines over coffee. I am woman hear me roar!'*

Lunchbox grids can be a real help for the busy family and especially if a few different people are responsible for packing children's lunches. The idea was born after seeing a Far Side comic strip of a mother standing in front of a large poster, holding a cooking pot. The poster showed a grid with children's names across the top and vegetables listed down the side. Under each child's name, alongside each food, was a comment such as '*loves it, likes it, hates it, tolerates it, throws it, allergic to it* [and] *projectile vomits it*'. The lunchbox grid is a nod to the fact that we are not all the same and that our differences make us unique. With days of the week along the top and children's names down the side, you can prepare a battle plan for the week's lunches. Your child should have some input into these grids as they are the end-user and most of the time out of your sight. You can use the same concept as dinner meal planning, to help guide them towards healthy options.

Not too far removed from boarding school concepts, children may also come to associate some foods with particular days of the week. Granted each day there will be a sandwich (fillings can change) and fruit, but Wednesday might be 'popcorn day' and Friday could be 'yoghurt day' or however else you'd like to mix it up. Making up all lunches and freezing them and any homemade baking ahead of time makes packing a lunchbox more like dealing out cards than drudgery in the early hours of the morning. Below you will find a pot of gold: a lunchbox grid with ten days' worth of balanced lunchboxes!

Table 24: Lunchbox grid—ten days of balanced lunchboxes

Day	Morning tea	Lunch	Afternoon tea
1	Crackers and hommus + apricots	Vegemite and cheese sandwich (wholegrain) + mandarin	Banana + celery, cheese and carrot
2	Yoghurt + grapes	Ham, tomato and cream cheese pita + carrot sticks	Apple + popcorn + milk
3	Pikelets + yoghurt drink	Chicken and avocado roll + dried apricots	Cheese wedges + nibblers
4	Custard + orange wedges	Cheesy asparagus fingers + watermelon	Banana + sultanas
5	Crackers and peanut paste + strawberries	Savoury frittata + cherry tomatoes	Yoghurt + grapes
6	Yoghurt + cereal + honey	Turkey and cranberry wheels + melon balls	Raisin bread + carrot sticks
7	Cheese wedges + watermelon	Egg and lettuce roll + mandarin	Yoghurt drink + popcorn
8	Crackers with cheese or jam + apple	Baked bean toasties + orange wedges	Hard-boiled egg + sultanas
9	Nibblers + milk	Tuna and cheese toasties + strawberries	Custard + watermelon
10	Melon balls + yoghurt drink	Tomato and hommus roll + apple	Pikelets + mandarin

Lunchbox grid—Putting it all together

Day 1

- Spread 3–4 crackers of choice with hommus + 3 dried apricots or 6 apricot halves.
- 2 slices bread with margarine, sliced cheese and Vegemite (to taste).
- Spreadable cream cheese, celery and carrot + Whole or chopped banana.

Day 2

- Choose pre-packed tub of yoghurt or place 100 g into a small container + A large handful of grapes (equals 1 serve).
- One small pita bread, spread with cream cheese, with slices of ham and tomato + Half a carrot diced, grated or cut into small strips.
- Pop corn in small amount of oil + Apple (cut or leave whole if preferred) + Regular milk dispensed into a container or pre-packed long-life milk (doesn't require refrigeration).

Day 3

- Try regular, mini or homemade pikelets, spread with margarine and jam of choice + There are a number of different brands of yoghurt drinks in varying flavours.
- One small dinner roll (white, grain or herb and garlic) with sliced chicken and avocado + A few dried apricots.
- Try a variety of different cheese wedges, slices or cubed cheese.

Day 4

- Use pre-packed custard or put 100 ml into a small container + Chop an orange into small wedges.
- Lightly toast bread, cut each slice into 3, spread with margarine, arrange 2 asparagus spears on each, top with cheese and grill until golden + Cut watermelon into triangles (leaving skin on if preferred).
- Cavendish or lady finger banana (chopped or left whole for child to peel) + Small handful of sultanas.

Day 5

- 2 cracker breads of choice spread with peanut paste or cashew paste + 2–3 large strawberries (chopped or left whole).
- Thinly slice 2 potatoes. Fry with finely chopped onion in small amount of oil. Add 2 chopped tomatoes, 1 cup of frozen peas and corn. Add 100 g chopped pre-cooked lean bacon, ham, meat or chicken of choice. Stir-fry for 2 minutes. Reduce heat. Beat 6 eggs and 2 tablespoons milk. Poor over cooked vegetables. Arrange 1 sliced avocado on top. Simmer slowly on low heat until almost set. Sprinkle with cheese and lightly brown under the grill. Serve with 3 cherry tomatoes.
- 100 g tub yoghurt + A large handful of grapes (preferably seedless).

Day 6

- Sprinkle crunchy cereal enriched with iron and other vitamins and minerals in with the yoghurt and honey or send separately for the children to mix (so it doesn't go soggy).
- Roll out bread (removing crusts), layer cream cheese, cranberry sauce and turkey (or chicken), roll into a log and cut into wheels + Try rockmelon, honeydew and watermelon balls.

Spread a slice of fruit bread or raisin bread with cream cheese and honey or jam of choice + Cut half a carrot into sticks.

Day 7

1 cheese wedge or stick or 20 g cheese of choice + 1 cup chopped or 2 triangles of watermelon.

Mash 1 hard-boiled egg with 1–2 tablespoons of mayonnaise or dijonnaise for flavour, tear or chop 1 medium lettuce leaf (try different flavours of lettuce), and arrange in small dinner roll + Peel or leave mandarin whole.

1 cup of home-popped (salt free) popcorn + Yoghurt drink of choice.

Day 8

Try different crackers or crispbreads spread with cream cheese and jam + 1 small apple or half a large (chopped or left whole).

Lightly spray a sandwich maker with spray oil. Place 4–5 tablespoons of baked beans on the bread. Baked beans come in a variety of flavours. Add a slice of cheese or 2 tablespoons of grated cheese on top of the baked beans. Cover with the second piece of bread and toast. Serve with an orange cut into wedges.

Place an egg in a saucepan of cold water and bring to the boil. Remove from heat and let sit in hot water for 12 minutes. Rinse with tap cool water and remove the shell. Serve with a handful of sultanas.

Day 9

Nibblers can be a selection of chopped fresh fruit and dried fruit, had with a glass of milk.

Spread plain or flavoured tuna on lightly toasted bread, sprinkle with grated cheese, grill till golden and cut into triangles + 2–3 large strawberries.

100 g tub custard + 1 cup of cubed watermelon.

Day 10

1 cup of cubed or balled melon (honeydew, rockmelon or watermelon) + Yoghurt drink of choice.

1 small dinner roll (white, multigrain or herb), spread with 1–2 tablespoons of hommus, with slices of tomato or cherry tomatoes + A small apple (cut into segments or leave whole).

4 mini or 2 large pikelets spread with cream cheese, jam or honey + 1 small mandarin (peeled).

About the authors

Kate writes ... I have always loved food and was blessed with a mother who was a fabulous cook. I can remember waking up in Canberra on cold winter mornings with the smell of lasagna or a three cheese spinach pie wafting down to my bedroom. My mother had been up since 5 a.m., showered, dressed and the evening meal already prepared eight hours in advance; talk about being organised.

The kitchen was the hub of our home. Everything was made from scratch even down to the jam made from the plums from our trees in the backyard (we had around 60 or so bottles to consume after every season!). So I guess it was just a natural progression for me to move into a career that enabled me to continuously discuss and help people with food preparation and menu planning. I have been an accredited practising dietitian for the past 16 years and I thought I knew it all, until I had children of my own. Having children has not only enriched my life but has enabled me to experience first hand the difficulties and pressures of finding and providing healthy interesting meals for the younger members of the family that we can all enjoy. It has also taught me that not everything runs to a schedule.

I was incredibly fortunate to marry a chef who brought the wonders of 'staring into an empty pantry and whipping up a storm' to my life—I'm still not sure how he does it! Food for our children, as you may guess, has always been full of flavour and full of 'surprises'. Yes, there has been anarchy on a number of nights; however, we have always stood united and stuck to our game plan when it came to serving up healthy foods for the family. In 2007 we worked together and published two cookbooks, *Kids Meals the Whole Family Will Love* and *Slimming and Health: Low fat summer cookbook*. My husband also helped me structure my website www.ultimatelunchbox.com.au

In my private practices in Brisbane I have seen hundreds of families with differing health needs, many with the common thread of a child with fussy eating tendencies. I have been specialising in family nutrition with a keen interest in fussy eating in children for the last ten years.

Meeting Julie in 2007 was like finding the final piece of the puzzle. I have now learned and understood so much more about why children can't chew, why they gag on food, will not mix foods together or will not move from a blended texture. Marrying our two professions has unlocked the secrets to successfully overcoming fussy eating practices.

I regularly discover parents who feel overwhelmed by all the things they read about what they should feed their children. This is why I put my hand up eight years ago for the position of media spokesperson for the Dietitians Association of Australia. I wanted to be involved in getting the right nutritional message out into the marketplace. To this end I have presented on shows such as *Brisbane Extra, Today* and *What's Good for You?* on Channel 9's *Sunrise*. I regularly consult to the corporate industry and have been involved in project media launches for companies such as Sunny Queen Farms, Subway Fresh Fit Australia, Yoplait, Little Tummy Tucker, Australian Bananas, Favco fresh apple slices and Kellogg's Australia. I have been writing regular nutritional columns for *Practical Parenting* magazine and regularly provide health stories for the *Sunday Mail* and magazines including *New Idea, Woman's Day* and *Good Health & Medicine*.

Julie writes . . . Growing up with one Australian and one European parent does much to dispel a child's fear of 'new and different' foods. Going to Nana's meant sausages and pomme potatoes, while a trip to Babcia's (Polish for 'grandma') meant mince and rice wrapped in cabbage leaves with a homemade tomato sauce, sauerkraut with onions, and lashings of creamy mashed potatoes. At Babcia's it was not possible to 'win' at dinnertime. If you left food on your plate there was the inquisition about what was wrong with the food. If you managed to eat the enormous plateful, surely she had not given you enough and more food would appear.

I did not learn to cook till I left home. My husband had better culinary skills having done a cooking course for boys at high school. Slowly and with some disasters I learned to cook from scratch using basic cookbooks. In 1999 I became 'Dr Julie' with a doctor of philosophy in chewing and swallowing (and the sounds you make when you swallow). I have degrees in psychology, linguistics and speech pathology. My husband is a dentist (but would have preferred to be a game-show host), so when the children arrived, we thought feeding them would be a breeze. As it turns out, our real education had only just begun. We have lived with reflux (we thought it was normal to smell of vomit and have a protector on the couch), fussy eating habits, enlarged tonsils, food texture and smell 'issues', an omnivore, a fabulous fruit bat, a meat-o-saurus and children who could not be bribed. In fact our youngest child's eating patterns marked the beginning of my journey into fussy eating and learning how to teach children to try new foods. He has been the guinea pig for many of the techniques successfully tried. Our older children have helped me to understand food from their perspective, and forced me to develop ways of explaining *why* they need to choose to eat healthy foods.

I have worked with adults and children with communication difficulties for 18 years, but for more for than 15 years I have worked clinically and conducted research into issues associated with eating, drinking, choking and pneumonia, from infants to the elderly. We take eating for granted as much as we take breathing for granted. People find it hard to understand that not everyone 'just chews and swallows food'. I love sharing this amazing world of eating by lecturing at universities, conferences and post-graduate workshops.

Currently I am working with cutting-edge researchers at the University of Queensland. I have been proud to be a consultant on swallowing difficulties for Speech Pathology Australia, the Dietitians Association of Australia, and the National Stroke Foundation. In 2009, I was humbled by an invitation to present to the International Dysphagia Research Society (swallowing disorders). I am an international author and reviewer of manuscripts for medical, nursing and allied health journals. I am also co-editor and author of the textbook *Dysphagia: Foundation, Theory and Practice* (2006).

Working with fussy eaters helped me to understand that I had part of the equation. I understand the biomechanics, anatomy and physiology of chewing and swallowing. I recognise the importance of food textures to chewing and swallowing. I appreciate food viewed through a child's eyes. What I didn't have was an understanding of hunger cycles, the roles of different nutrients, essential servings of food groups, portion sizes, et cetera. Meeting Kate provided me with a key to a fantastic new place; an '*Ah-ha*' moment. Our complementary approach helps to make sense of the fussy eater puzzle, no matter what age.

Appendix

Explanatory notes and tables

Note that the largest weight gains per day happen in the first six months of life. Boys and girls have different growth velocities (speeds of growth). Note differences in weight gain around the time of puberty. These charts provide an *average* for weight gain. Each person is an individual and should have their own weight monitored using child health record books. Note also that weight must be taken in the context of the person's height. Parental height will affect the eventual height of their children. Children who are acutely unwell with a cold, flu or diarrhoea may show a temporary decrease in food intake. This is quite normal and children will generally increase their appetite once they have recovered. Children who remain unwell and underweight or have chronic poor growth should be referred to their local doctor or paediatrician. For example, children with chronic failure to thrive may show low iron levels, reduced food intake, malabsorption of nutrients and stunted growth.

On the following pages are two tables that show expected weight gains for boys and girls with month-by-month averages for the first year and then yearly weight gains till children are 18 years.

Table 25: Expected weight gains per year for boys[1,2]

Age	Average weight (kg)	Average weight gain per day (g)	Average weight gain per year (kg)
1 month	4.58	35.2	
2 months	5.5	30.4	
3 months	6.28	23.2	
4 months	6.94	19.1	
5 months	7.48	16.1	
6 months	7.93	12.8	
7 months	8.3	11.0	
8 months	8.62	10.4	
9 months	8.89	9.0	
10 months	9.13	7.9	
11 months	9.37	7.7	
12 months	9.62	8.2	
1 year–1 year 9 months	11.5	6.6	2.4
2 years to 2 years 9 months	13.5	5.5	2.0
3 years to 3 years 9 months	15.7	5.8	2.1
4 years to 4 years 9 months	17.7	5.5	2.0
5 years to 5 years 9 months	19.7	5.5	2.0
6 years to 6 years 9 months	21.7	6.0	2.2
7 years to 7 years 9 months	24.0	6.6	2.4
8 years to 8 years 9 months	26.7	7.7	2.8
9 years to 9 years 9 months	29.7	9.0	3.3
10 years to 10 years 9 months	33.3	10.7	3.9
11 years to 11 years 9 months	37.5	12.3	4.5
12 years to 12 years 9 months	42.3	14.2	5.2
13 years to 13 years 9 months	47.8	15.9	5.8
14 years to 14 years 9 months	53.8	16.2	5.9
15 years to 15 years 9 months	59.5	14.8	5.4
16 years to 16 years 9 months	64.4	11.5	4.2
17 years to 17 years 9 months	67.8	7.1	2.6

Table 26: **Expected weight gains per year for girls**[1,2]

Age	Average weight (kg)	Average weight gain per day (g)	Average weight gain per year (kg)
1 month	4.35	28.3	
2 months	5.14	25.5	
3 months	5.82	21.2	
4 months	6.41	18.4	
5 months	6.92	15.5	
6 months	7.35	12.8	
7 months	7.71	11.0	
8 months	8.03	9.2	
9 months	8.31	8.4	
10 months	8.55	7.7	
11 months	8.78	6.6	
12 months	9.0	6.3	
1 year–1 year 9 months	10.8	6.6	2.4
2 years to 2 years 9 months	13.0	6.0	2.2
3 years to 3 years 9 months	15.1	5.2	1.9
4 years to 4 years 9 months	16.8	4.7	1.7
5 years to 5 years 9 months	18.6	4.9	1.8
6 years to 6 years 9 months	20.6	6.3	2.3
7 years to 7 years 9 months	23.3	8.2	3.0
8 years to 8 years 9 months	26.6	10.1	3.7
9 years to 9 years 9 months	30.5	11.0	4.0
10 years to 10 years 9 months	34.7	12.3	4.5
11 years to 11 years 9 months	39.2	12.3	4.5
12 years to 12 years 9 months	43.8	12.6	4.6
13 years to 13 years 9 months	48.3	11.5	4.2
14 years to 14 years 9 months	52.1	9.3	3.4
15 years to 15 years 9 months	55.0	6.0	2.2
16 years to 16 years 9 months	56.4	2.2	0.8
17 years to 17 years 9 months	56.7	0	0

My child's food history

Use this template (with examples) to track your child's diet. Complete the diet history for a week (if you're really pushed for time, two weekdays and a weekend should cover it). Aim to re-do the diet history six to 12 months after you've started implementing the suggested changes. An example of a completed profile is included below. A blank profile is also included below (Table 28).

Table 27: Example of a child's food history

Day: Friday 13th March, 2009				
Time of day	How long did the meal/snack take?	What was offered?	Of what was offered, how much was eaten?	Notes: food texture, food groups covered, food groups missing, meals offered every 2–3 hours?
7 a.m.	25 minutes	Bowl of Nutrigrain with ½ cup of milk, 1 glass of milk, 1 piece of toast	Half bowl of cereal, no toast, all milk	Lots of soft and dissolvable foods here (minimal chewing required). A very unbalanced diet. At risk for nutrient deficiencies. Milk and dairy overload, but almost no iron (eg. red meat, etc.). Poor fruit intake, no vegetables.
10.30 a.m.	10 minutes	Tub of apple puree, tub of custard, 1 slice of cheese, 1 packet chips, 1 peanut butter sandwich	Half apple puree, all custard, all cheese, all chips, one bite of sandwich	
3 p.m.	10 minutes	1 bowl of two-minute noodles, 1 chocolate wafer	All noodles, all chocolate wafer	

Time of day	How long did the meal/snack take?	What was offered?	Of what was offered, how much was eaten?	Notes: food texture, food groups covered, food groups missing, meals offered every 2–3 hours?
4 p.m.	5 minutes	1 tub of custard 6 savoury crackers	All custard All crackers	Minimal cereals or grains.
6 p.m.	1 hour	1 slice shepherd's pie, salad	One bite of pie, no salad	Big gap between morning tea and next meal offering.
8 p.m.	5 minutes	Small tin spaghetti and ice block	All spaghetti and ice block	Dinnertime is too long.

Table 28: **My child's food history**

Day				
Time of day	How long did the meal/snack take?	What was offered?	Of what was offered, how much was eaten?	Notes: food texture, food groups covered, food groups missing, meals offered every 2-3 hours?

Notes

Chapter 1 Developmental stages of eating

1. Guiding principles for complementary feeding of the breastfed child. 2003, World Health Organization.
2. Prescott, S.L., Tang, M.L.K. and Bjorksten, B. 2007, Primary allergy prevention in children: Updated summary of a position statement of the Australasian Society of Clinical Immunology and Allergy. *Medical Journal of Australia*. Position statement.
3. Berzlanovich, A.M., Muhm, M., Sim, E. *et al.* 1999, Foreign body asphyxiation: An autopsy study. *The American Journal of Medicine*, vol. 107, pp. 351–355.
4. Bren, L. 2005, Prevent your child from choking. *FDA Consumer*, vol 39, no. 5, pp. 27–30 (Sept/Oct).
5. Carruth, B.R. and Skinner, J.D. 2002, Feeding behaviour and other motor development in healthy children (2–24 months). *Journal of the American College of Nutrition* vol. 21, no. 2, pp. 88–96.
6. Center for Disease Control and Prevention. 2001, Non-fatal choking related episodes among children, United States. *Morbidity and Mortality Weekly Report*, vol. 51, pp. 945–948.
7. Morley, R.E., Ludemann, J.P., Moxham, J.P. *et al.* 2004, Foreign body aspiration in infants and toddlers: Recent trends in British Columbia. *The Journal of Otolaryngology*, vol. 33, no. 1, pp. 37–41.
8. Mu, L., Ping, H. and Sun, D. 1991, Inhalation of foreign bodies in Chinese children: A review of 400 cases. *Laryngoscope*, vol. 101, pp. 657–660.

9. Rimmell, F., Thome, A., Stool, S., *et al.* 1995, Characteristics of objects that cause choking in children. *JAMA*, vol. 274, no. 22, Dec 13, pp. 1763–1766.

10. Wolach, B., Raz, A., Weinberg, J. *et al.* 1994, Aspirated bodies in the respiratory tract of children: Eleven years experience with 127 patients. *International Journal of Pediatric Otorhinolaryngology*, vol. 30, pp. 1–10.

Chapter 2   Surviving the age of typical food fussiness (18 months–3½ years)

1. Hausner, H., Bredie, W.L.P, Molgaard, C., Petersen, M.A., Moller, P. 2008, Differential transfer of dietary compounds into human breast milk. *Physiology & Behaviour*, vol. 95 (issue 1–2), pp. 118–124.

2. Mannella, J.A. and Beauchamp, J.K. 1991, Maternal diet alters the sensory qualities of human milk and the nursling's behaviour. *Pediatrics*, vol. 88, pp. 737–744.

3. Butte, N. 2005, Energy requirements of infants. *Public Health Nutrition*, vol. 8, no. 7A, pp. 953–967.

4. Torun, B. 2005, Energy requirements for children and adolescents. *Public Health Nutrition*, vol. 8, no. 7A, pp. 968–993.

5. Kasese-Hara, M., Wright, C. and Drewett, R. 2002, Energy compensation in young children who fail to thrive. *Journal of Child Psychology and Psychiatry*, vol. 43, no. 4, pp. 449–456.

6. Cooke. L., Wardle, J. and Gibson, E.L. 2003, Relationship between parental report of food neophobia and everyday food consumption in 2–6-year-old children. *Appetite*, vol. 41, pp. 205–206.

7. Johnson, S.L. 2002, Children's food acceptance patterns: The interface of ontogency and nutrition needs. *Nutrition Review*, vol. 60, no. 5, pp. S91–S94.

8. Nicklaus, S., Boggio, V. and Issanchou, S. 2005, Food choices at lunch during the third year of life: High selection of animal and starchy foods but avoidance of vegetables. *Acta Paediatrica*, vol. 94 pp. 943–951.

9. Nicklaus, S., Boggio, V., Chanabet, C. and Issanchou, S. 2005, A prospective study of food variety seeking in childhood, adolescence and early adult life. *Appetite*, vol. 44, pp. 289–297.

Chapter 4   I've got a 'fussy eater', now what?

1. Hoebler, C., Devaux, M-F., Karinthi, A., Belleville, C., Barry, J-L. 2000, Particle size of solid food after human mastication and in vitro simultation of oral breakdown. *International Journal of Food Sciences and Nutrition*, vol. 51, pp. 353–366.

Chapter 5   Medical reasons for food refusal

1. McIntyre, G.T. and McIntyre, G.M. 2002, Teething troubles? *British Dental Journal*, vol. 192, no. 5, pp. 251–255.
2. Dental care for babies and young children—Fact sheet. 2007, Australian Dental Association: Mi-tech Medical Publishing (www.mitec.com.au).
3. Wake, M., Hesketh, K. and Allen, M.A. 1999, Parent beliefs about infant teething: A survey of Australian parents. *Journal of Paediatrics and Child Health*, vol. 35, pp. 446–449.
4. Holloway, R.H. and Orenstein, S.R. 1991, Gastro-oesophageal reflux disease in adults and children. *Bailliere's Clinical Gastroenterology*, vol. 5, no. 2, pp. 337–370.
5. Watson Genna, C. 2008, *Supporting sucking skills in breastfeeding infants*. Jones and Bartlett Publishers, Boston.
6. Morgan, A. and Reilly, S. 2006, 'Clinical signs, aetiologies and characteristics of paediatric dysphagia' in J. Cichero and B. Murdoch (eds), *Dysphagia: Foundation, theory and practice*. John Wiley & Sons Ltd., Chichester, pp. 391–465.
7. Duca, A.P., Dantas, R.O., Rodrigues, A.A.C. and Sawamura, R. 2008, Evaluation of swallowing in children with vomiting after feeding. *Dysphagia*, vol. 23, pp. 177–182.

8. Dualibi, A.P.F.F., Pignatari, S.S.H. and Weckx, L.L.W. 2002, Nutritional evaluation in surgical treatment of children with hypertrophic tonsils and adenoids. *International Journal of Pediatric Otorhinolaryngology*, vol. 66, no. 2, pp. 107–113.

For further information regarding tonsils and adenoids, please visit www.betterhealth.vic.gov.au

Chapter 7 The 'rules of engagement': Rules at mealtimes

1. Smeets, A.J.P.G. and Westerterp-Plantenga, M.S. 2006, Oral exposure and sensory-specific satiety. *Physiology & Behaviour*, vol. 89, pp. 281–286.
2. Case-Smith, J. 2005, *Occupational therapy for children*, 2nd edition, Elsevier, St Louis.
3. Evans Morris, S. and Dunn Klein, M. 2000, *Pre-Feeding Skills*, 2nd edition, US, Therapy Skill Builders.
4. Galloway, A.T., Fiorito, L.M., Francis, L.A. and Birch, L.L. 2006, 'Finish your soup': Counterproductive effects of pressuring children to eat on intake and affect. *Appetite*, vol. 46, pp. 318–323.
5. Noble, G., Stead, M., Jones, S., McDermott, L., McVie, D. 2007, The paradoxical food buying behaviour of parents: Insights from the UK and Australia. *British Food Journal*, vol. 109, no. 5, pp. 387–398.
6. Nicklaus, S., Boggio, V. and Issanchou, S. 2005, Food choices at lunch during the third year of life: High selection of animal and starchy foods but avoidance of vegetables. *Acta Paediatric*, vol. 94, pp. 943–951.

Chapter 8 Surviving the older child

1. Monneuse, M-O., Rigal, N., Frelut, M-L., Hladik, C-M., Simmen, B. and Pasquet, P. 2008, Taste acuity of obese adolescents and changes in food neophobia and food preferences during a weight reduction session. *Appetite*, vol. 50, pp. 302–307.

2.	Birch, L.L. 1998, Psychological influences on the childhood diet. *The Journal of Nutrition*, vol. 128, no. 2S, pp. 407S–410S.

3.	Australian National Children's Nutrition and Physical Activity Survey. 2007, Australian Government Department of Health & Aging; Australian Food and Grocery Council; Australian Government Department of Agriculture, Fisheries and Forestry.

4.	Nicklaus, S., Boggio, B., Chabanet, C., Issanchou, S. 2005, A prospective study of food variety seeking in childhood, adolescence and early adult life. *Appetite*, vol. 44, pp. 289–297.

5.	Healthy Kids Queensland Survey. 2006, Queensland Government, Queensland Health, University of Queensland.

6.	New South Wales Schools Physical Activity and Nutrition Survey, 2004.

7.	Lewindon, P. 2007, *Eating Disorders*. Children's Nutrition Research Centre Conference. Brisbane, 30 April–1 May 2007.

8.	Hark, L. and Deen, D. 2007, *Nutrition: The definitive Australian guide to eating for good health*. Dorling Kindersley Australasia Pty. Ltd., Melbourne.

Chapter 9   Tips for shopping, cooking, lunchboxes and others

1.	Edwards, J.S.A. and Hartwell, H.H. 2002, Fruit and vegetables: Attitudes and knowledge of primary school children. *Journal of Human Nutrition and Dietetics*, vol. 15, no. 5, pp. 365–374.

2.	Hendy, H.M. and Raudenbush, B. 2000, Effectiveness of teacher modelling to encourage food acceptance in preschool children. *Appetite*, vol. 34, pp. 61–76.

Appendix

1.	Butte, N.F. 2005, Energy requirements of infants. *Public Health Nutrition*, vol. 8, no. 7a, pp. 953–967.

2.	Torun, B. 2005, Energy requirements of children and adolescents. *Public Health Nutrition*, vol. 8, no. 7a, pp. 968–993.